The New Approach to Cancer

by Cameron Stauth

English Brothers Press
New York
Book Division Representatives:
Health News Media, Box 2186, Eugene, Oregon 97402
1-800-547-8995

The New Approach to Cancer

This book is not intended as medical advice; it should not be used in lieu of a doctor's treatment. Any person who is in ill health should visit his or her doctor.

ISBN No. 0-942686-01-2

First Printing April 1982

Library of Congress No. 82-50176

Cover design and illustration by Carol Salvin

YOU CAN FIGHT CANCER YOU CAN BE IN CONTROL

Recovery from cancer is occurring increasingly often — partly because patients are taking an active role in fighting the disease.

You need not be a passive, helpless cancer "victim." You can help your doctor conquer cancer by stimulating your own health. This is *the new approach to cancer.*

It is an approach that has been pioneered by Dr. William Donald Kelley and his colleagues.

In this book you will find a full description of the program of health stimulation that has helped thousands of people. For over twenty years, Dr. Kelley has taught doctors how to help their patients recover.

Now you can learn how yourself.

YOU CAN STOP BEING AFRAID OF CANCER

Dedication

This book is dedicated to Doctor William Donald Kelley, in appreciation for his exceptional concern about other people.

It is also dedicated to the doctors at Sloan-Kettering Institute and other technologically-oriented physicians, in appreciation for the sacrifices they have had to make to master their skills.

Finally, and not least importantly, the book is dedicated to Shari Ann Levine, as a modest token of appreciation for the many gifts she has given.

About the Author

Cameron Stauth is a journalist specializing in health science reporting. He is former editor-in-chief of *Eugene Magazine, The Journal of the Nutritional Academy, The Journal of Health Science* and *The International Health Institute letter.* He is co-author of the books *Folk Medicine for Today* (Rodale Press, publishers of *Prevention* magazine), *The Starch-Blocker Cookbook* (T. S. Vernon and Sons), *The Starch Blocker Diet,* and is author of *The New Approach to Cancer.* He is author of many magazine articles, has won several journalistic awards, is a former hospital public relations director, is founder of the Cancer Prevention Society, and hosts a television health program.

Acknowledgements

The author would like to express sincere appreciation to all of the people who helped create this book. Nancy Smith helped a great deal in the early stages of the book with typing, secretarial and organizational work, and Roberta Hinds, who also did the index and proofreading, helped out in the latter stages. Colleen Costen-Murff obtained all of the releases for publication from other publishers, and Comp/Graphics typeset it. David Dinerman provided considerable advice and support, and David Stauth and David Shaw took care of business during the writing of the book. My friends at the I.H.I., including Kim and Rita, provided encouragement. The author would also like to thank Mary Ann and my other friends at the Wild Iris cafe, where most of this book was written, for proving on a daily basis that health-providing food can also be delicious.

Table of Contents

The publisher would like to express appreciation for reprint permissions from the following:

J. P. Tarcher, *Getting Well Again,* by O. Carl Simonton, M.D., Stephanie Matthews-Simonton and James Creighton.

Houghton Mifflin Company. From *The Cancer Connection* by Larry Agran. Copyright ©1977 by Larry Agran. Reprinted by permission of Houghton Mifflin Company.

Random House, *Conquering Cancer,* by Lucien Israel, M.D., translated by Joan Pinkham, copyright ©1979 by Lucien Israel.

W. W. Norton and Company, Inc., *Preventing Cancer,* by Elizabeth Whelan, Ph.D.

Linus Pauling Institute of Science and Medicine, *Cancer and Vitamin C,* by Linus Pauling.

Keats Publishing Company, from the book *Cancer and Its Nutritional Therapies,* by Richard A. Passwater, Ph.D., copyright ©1978 by Richard A. Passwater, Ph.D. Reprinted by permission of Keats Publishing, Inc., New Canaan, CT.

W. Marshall Ringsdorf Jr., D.M.D., from *Diet and Disease,* by Cheraskin and Ringsdorf.

Grove Press, *The Cancer Syndrome,* by Ralph Moss. Reprinted by permission of Grove Press, Inc. Copyright ©1980 by Ralph Moss.

Yale University Press, for *Man Adapting* by Rene Dubos.

Prentice-Hall, Inc., for *Cancer: How to Prevent It and How to Help Your Doctor Fight It,* by George Berkley, Ph.D., ©1978 by Prentice-Hall, Inc., Englewood Cliffs, NJ 07632.

PART ONE

Cancer Is A Personal Affair

The people will live on.
The learning and blundering people will live on.
They will be tricked and sold and again sold
And go back to the nourishing earth for rootholds.
The people, so peculiar in renewal and comeback,
You can't laugh off their capacity to take it.

—Carl Sandburg

CHAPTER ONE

What You Don't Know

Many signs tell you that you have cancer, but likely as not you do not see them, because people generally don't see what they are afraid to see.

Being called back by your doctor for further, follow-up x-rays is one sign that something is wrong. If the doctor himself, rather than a nurse or orderly, wheels you down to the x-ray room, that should be a sign to you that something out of the ordinary is happening. You would think, if you were being totally logical, "He must be taking me himself so that he can tell me something in private." If you were being absolutely rational, you could see, as he wheels your chair into the elevator, the tight worried look on his face, and know that it is a bad sign.

When the elevator doors seal the two of you off from the rest of the hospital, you would, if you were being realistic, wait for the doctor to say, "I'm sorry, but the initial x-rays didn't look good. Every indication at this point is that you do have cancer." If it were a television show you were watching — a soap opera, perhaps — you would expect these words to come from the doctor. But if it is real life, your own life, you don't expect them.

But this verdict should come as no shock to you, because you have probably had symptoms of ill health for some time. You may have found a bump or a lump or a sore spot or a peculiar growth on the surface of your skin. You may have felt tired and weak for several months, or even several years, even though you have been getting enough sleep. Your emotions may have been undependable of late, casting you into depression one day and into an uncharacteristic display of temper the next. You may have developed a cough, or chronic indigestion, for the first time in your life. Maybe you have lost some weight recently, even though your eating habits have been the same as always.

Some problems, whatever they are, have probably developed with your health, problems that prompted you to consult with your physician. You may have been worried by these health problems, or, on the other hand, you may have regarded them with nonchalance.

If cancer has already struck people you are close to, though — particularly blood relatives — you probably haven't been able to be casual about your health problems. You may have told yourself you were just being a hypochondriac, but you probably thought of a relative's suffering and eventual death when your own health problems cropped up. That memory may have caused a stab of coldness to slice right through your body. But then you probably thought, "No, not me. I'll never get cancer.

Even when you're alone with the doctor in the elevator, knowing that preliminary x-rays have already been done, knowing that the doctor is worried about something, knowing that he wants to talk to you alone, you *still* don't believe he will tell you, in only a moment, that you have cancer.

You know he might deliver that verdict, though — you can't deny that there is a chance — so you sit silently in your wheelchair, as the elevator descends to the x-ray room in the basement, and wait for him to speak.

When he does speak, you feel as if he is talking to someone else, even though the two of you are alone.

It is mid-day, mid-July, hot outside and cool inside, in a quiet Long Island neighborhood. Robin Fonwood* waits for her doctor to call. He has already called once, promising to call back if he finds out the results of the preliminary, initial x-rays that had been taken of Robin. Her twin sister, Marie, who lives next door, and her 11-year-old daughter, Dora, wait with her. Robin and Marie cannot help but be worried. Robin's health has been bad for several years, bad enough for her doctor to recommend diagnostic x-rays. She has suffered from a severe cough, a lump in her throat,

*To protect privacy, the publisher has chosen to use fictitious names of patients and family members in this section. All locations and names of hospitals are real. All situations are actual and real.

chronic fatigue, recent weight loss, and depression. Both women, who are 34, know that their family has a history of cancer, and they can't help but think about the toll the disease has taken as they await the return call from the doctor.

They both remember the suffering of their brother, Tim, who had come down with cancer when he was 15. He had had Hodgkin's disease, a cancer of the lymphatic system, and had shrunk into an emaciated skeleton in about a year and a half. When the family had known he was going to die, they had brought him home from the hospital and had put his bed in the living room. There he had spent his last days, gaunt and groaning, nauseous and unable to eat, resting fitfully. His own immune system could no longer fight infection, because of the stresses of his disease and its treatments — toxic chemotherapy and radiation — so he was covered with infectious sores. He had become dependent upon pain-killing narcotics and was often so dazed by their effects that he was unaware of other people in the room.

As he slowly died, the 6'1'', formerly powerful young man became a dehumanized scarecrow that frightened his twin sisters.

Other deaths, equally as sad and ugly, followed. About a year before Robin began to have serious health problems, one uncle had died of lung cancer and another had died of lymphoma. An aunt had died of breast cancer, and Robin's mother had contracted breast cancer but survived. Two cousins had developed cancer, and a cousin's six-year-old son was struck by leukemia. Because Robin came from a large family, certain family members could be expected to eventually have cancer, since one in every four Americans contracts it. But the rate in her family was higher than the national average, causing all of them to have a special fear of the disease.

No one knew why Robin's family seemed especially vulnerable to cancer. They had all grown up on Long Island, and almost all the family members had stayed there. As a family, they had all been exposed to high doses of toxic pesticides that were regularly sprayed onto a nearby field, and had all grown up near one of America's first nuclear power plants. They had virtually all adopted careless diets, high in fatty and processed foods, and many family members had a slight tendency to be overweight. Otherwise, though, they were exposed to no greater degree of cancer risk factors than the average American family. Among themselves, they speculated that perhaps they had a genetic tendency toward cancer.

Robin, unlike some other members of the family, had a history of frequent use of birth control pills. She had taken them for many years, once for four consecutive years. She had also suffered a recent traumatic accident, a bad fall on an icy sidewalk that had injured her coccyx, which had seemed to weaken her constitution.

Even before the fall, though, which occurred in the early months of 1978, she had been suffering from poor health. Since 1973, she had endured chronic bronchitis, often so severe that she was confined to bed. About the same time she fell, she began to wheeze almost all the time, and was so tired that she was unable to do housework. She started to feel a lump in her throat when she swallowed. Her mood, generally cheerful and stable, began to be plagued by depression and anger. For the first time since the birth of her two children, she began to lose her temper with them. She would experience a fever for about two days every two weeks. By mid-1978, shortly before she consulted her doctor about her failing health, she was unable to climb the stairs of her home without resting afterwards for about 20 minutes. The feeling of having a lump in her throat intensified. Subtle changes occurred in her body, such as increased brittleness in her nails and extra oiliness and curliness in her hair. She became extremely vulnerable to viral infections, developing cold or flu symptoms almost every other week.

The days that she felt well — vibrant and strong, as she had for most of her life — dwindled. It occurred to her one day in June of 1978 that she *never* felt well anymore. Not once in a while — not ever.

She went to her doctor and asked for a complete physical exam. "Robin," he told her, "if I gave a physical to all the healthy people who thought they needed one, I wouldn't have time for sick people." He told her, in an abrupt, almost abusive way, that all her health problems would be solved if she would just lose 10 pounds of weight — strange advice, she felt, since weight loss was one of her recent problems. His attitude, condescending and cold, did not particularly anger her, because she was not in the habit of getting angry at people. Nor was she particularly disturbed about having visited a member of the medical profession without having had her medical problems solved. Because she had witnessed the medical community's inability to help her relatives, she harbored few illusions about doctors' abilities to solve all health problems at all times. Therefore, she decided to just endure her problems and wait for them to go away.

Her husband, however, *was* angry at her doctor's refusal to take her problems seriously. A successful building contractor in a highly competitive region, Mark Fonwood, aggressive and independent, insisted she consult another doctor.

So Robin Fonwood visited a young practitioner affiliated with Long Island's Good Samaritan Hospital, who told her that a full physical, including some chest x-rays, would be a good idea.

After the initial x-rays and several other tests, Robin Fonwood was sent home, having been told that the doctor would call if there were any serious problems. It was 30 days before the young doctor called; he had been on vacation and the x-ray had lain idly on the desk of his partner, who had never looked at it. The young doctor called her to say it looked as if more x-rays were needed, and that he would call her later in the day to tell her when to come in to the hospital.

Robin sits in her living room and waits for the doctor's second call. Her sister, a very frequent visitor, has come over to help her pass the time. They sit and talk for several hours, and the phone does not ring. Both of them think about cancer in the family as they wait. But neither mentions it.

The phone rings.

It is Robin's doctor (at the publisher's request, names of physicians have been deleted). "Robin," he says, "I think it would be best if you would come in for more x-rays as soon as you can."

"Tomorrow is Friday," she says. "Can I come in the first part of next week?"

"I think you should come in tomorrow." She feels panic rise, but pushes it down.

"What did the x-rays show?"

"We can't be sure until we do more."

"Doctor," she says, "whatever it is, I want you to tell me about it as soon as you know."

The doctor tells her that he will, and schedules her for tests the next morning. When she hangs up, she tells Marie as casually as she can, that they want to do more tests. Marie replies, as casually as she can, that more tests are probably a good idea, because they will help the doctors figure out once and for all what's wrong, so that it can be fixed.

That evening, Robin calls her husband, who is working out of town, and tells him that by tomorrow they should know what is wrong. He tells her that he is going to return home immediately, and she doesn't protest. Before she goes to sleep, she becomes very frightened, and cries.

Mark Fonwood stands by his wife's hospital bed, chatting with her. The surgeon who supervised the second series of x-rays enters the room, tells Mark that the x-rays should be ready, and invites him to look at them with him.

Mark stands before the machine that dries the x-rays, shifting from foot to foot. The surgeon pulls the first x-ray out and clips it onto a viewing screen. He stiffens, and blurts out, before he can stop himself, "Oh, my God, this is no job for a surgeon." Mark feels his chest tighten as the doctor holds his fist against a dark mass that blemishes the x-ray of Robin's chest. "If that mass was the size of my fist," he says, "it would be difficult to remove, but possible." But the edges of the dark mass are clearly visible even with the doctor's fist directly over them.

Mark takes a breath and says calmly, "How long can a patient with a tumor that size live?"

"If a tumor is a form of Hodgkins disease, maybe eight to ten years, with chemotherapy," the doctor says. "If it's lymphoma, four to eight months with treatment. Based on how the lymph nodes in her neck felt, and the fact that her brother had Hodgkins, I'd say it's Hodgkins.

"In the morning," the doctor says, "we'll do a biopsy and find out which it is."

"Is there anything to do in the meantime?"

"No. Just pray it's Hodgkins."

Mark tells Robin that the x-rays are inconclusive, and that they need to do a biopsy to determine if she has a cyst, or a benign growth, "or whatever." She has prepared herself for conclusive news, good or bad, and is exasperated to be left up in the air again. "How long does it take them to find out what's wrong with you?"

she asks.

Mark notices her referring to herself as "you," a habit she is to engage in for many months. It comforts her to refer to herself in the third person, as if events were happening to someone else.

"Well, you can't blame them for wanting to be positive before they say what it is," Mark says.

"I think I have it," Robin says.

"Have what?"

"You know. Cancer."

"You don't know what you have, Robin. We'll just have to wait and see what they say." He feels sorry for her, lying passively against the clean white sheets. She has not even been diagnosed yet, and already, he thinks, she looks like "a whipped pup."

The biopsy does not reveal immediately if the cancer is Hodgkins or lymphoma. Samples have to be sent to Stony Brook University, which is affiliated with Good Samaritan Hospital. For several days, from July 7, 1978, to July 10, they wait.

Robin begins to show symptoms of "pre-vena cava syndrome," including a bulging of the eyes, which is caused by a blockage of the artery that returns blood from the head to the heart. The tumor in Robin's upper chest is also pressing against her trachea, or wind-pipe, making breathing difficult.

Robin's doctor, a young, bearded man not long out of his internship, is worried that she will die of asphyxiation or possibly circulatory blockage if the tumor is not shrunk almost immediately with radiation therapy. He feels that this step should be taken while they wait to see what kind of cancer it is, and how far advanced it has become.

"But if you do radiation on her," argues Robin's father in a conference with the doctor and Mark, "she'll know she has cancer, and I don't think she should know until we know what kind it is."

The brief controversy is abruptly ended by the arrival of the pathology report from Stony Brook.

It is hystiocytic lymphoma — the worst of all possibilities. The young doctor meets with Mark alone and tells him that his wife has eight to ten months to live, if she undergoes the unpleasant treatments of radiation and chemotherapy. With no therapy, he says, she might live four or five months. In any case, there is no longer any reason to delay the emergency radiotherapy that will temporarily shrink the tumor. The doctor goes to get Robin, to take her down to the radiology room, and to tell her that she will soon die. He tells Mark that he will tell her on the way down, and asks Mark to be waiting outside the elevator on the radiology floor.

She should have known, she later realized, that something was wrong when the doctor himself, and not her nurse, wheeled her to the elevator. She should have known by the look on his face that bad news was coming.

She has had time to prepare herself for the worst, but, when it comes time to hear it, she is not ready.

Her first question: "How long do I have?"

"It could be as long as eight to ten years," he tells her, "and by then they may have a cure for cancer." The doctor knows that if she is totally unprepared to accept her death, she will fasten onto this extremely optimistic maximum life possibility and will not ask about more realistic possibilities.

Her second question: "Doctor, if I had something very important do do, how soon should I do it?"

This is a hard question for him, and the young doctor, who has thus far worked with very few terminally ill patients, is almost crying when he answers it. "If you have something very important to do, Robin, you should try to do it in eight to ten months."

She knows. She feels icy, and can suddenly see all of herself, sitting in a wheelchair in an elevator, as if she is outside of her own body. She doesn't cry.

When the doors of the elevator open, Mark is there, and when he begins to cry, she does, too, and the doctor leaves them alone.

CHAPTER TWO

Doctor's Orders

When you are told that you will soon die, you wonder what it will be like. Suddenly a great intangible, unknowable event in your life — the occurrence of your death — becomes tangible; you can speculate with some accuracy how it will happen and where you will be when it happens.

If your death is being caused by a disease associated with pain and torment, you can become fixated on *how* you will die — thoughts of the manner of your death are never really gone, even when you are talking about something else or reading or watching television.

Doctors may give you Valium or sleeping pills or mood elevators, but these chemicals are no substitute for what you crave — a future like that of other people, one that may hold suffering but also may hold pleasure: a mysterious, unpredictable future. Sometimes you daydream about still having a future that is not medically predictable. You try not to daydream, though, because waking up from these daydreams is painful.

If you have seen other people die of the same disease you have, you wonder if you will die like they did. You wonder, if you have cancer, if you will become a skeleton in your bed, unable to hold food down, bald, and as physically helpless as an infant. You wonder if you will be brave, or if you will reach a point where you stop caring about your dignity and about maintaining the special threads of your personality and intellect that have always made you unique.

You wonder if any parts of your body will be cut away, and how you will look afterwards. You wonder if you will feel differently about yourself after surgery, or if other people will treat you differently.

You can't help but speculate what it will be like when you finally die — if that moment will have a special quality, or if it will be so surrounded with pain that you don't even notice it. You wonder if you will have time to say goodbye to your family, and if you do, you wonder what you will say. You wonder if the moment of your death will be welcome when it comes.

If you have strong religious beliefs, you try to imagine what your after-life will be like — if it will be closely connected to your life thus far, or if it will be so different that it is beyond your comprehension. If you are lucky, you don't have any doubts about whether or not there will be an after-life.

You think about your family and friends all the time. Sometimes you see your death as an instrument of hurt against them, and you are almost angry at yourself for doing it to them. You try to devise ways to help them accept your being gone. But if you have young children, you can't help but despair, because you know there is really no way to shield them. If you have had problems with your husband or mother or close friend — and who hasn't? — you try to think of ways to work things out while there is still time.

Often, you start out thinking about your death, and then you begin thinking about the illness that is causing it, and that makes you think about what you have gone through that day to treat the illness, and what you will have to go through the next day.

If what you have to go through the next day will hurt, you dread it, and, as you look out your window in the middle of the night, you wonder if the treatments, and the continuation of life that they bring, are worth the hurt. If you are going to die, shouldn't you just get ready to die?

Robin's roommate at Good Samaritan asks to have another room, because she hears Robin is dying of cancer. Mark needs to be home most of the time to take care of the kids, Dora and little Jimmy, so Robin is alone much of the time, and is alone all night, often unable to sleep. She watches automobile headlights move by outside her window for hours, and her mind wanders.

Often she worries about her family. One of the first things that she thought, when her doctor told her that she had only four to eight months to live, was that her twin sister, Marie, would soon have her first birthday alone. She knows her death will devastate her twin sister — who is also her next-door neighbor and best friend — and that it will make her entire extended family miserable. She worries mostly about her children, though, who are both still in grade school. The first thing she said to Mark as they cried outside the elevator was, "What am I going to tell the children?" As the certainty of her death sinks in, she finds that she doesn't worry too much about Mark, because she knows he can take care of himself. But she knows the children can't.

Therefore, Robin lies awake at night, trying to comprehend what is happening to her, imagining what will happen to her in the future, and attempting to find solutions to problems that do not have solutions.

Mark, through force of his own will, is able to have Robin admitted to New York City's Sloan-Kettering Memorial Hospital, the foremost cancer treatment facility in the world. Her admission to the facility is discouraged by the doctors at Sloan-Kettering, on the grounds that she is a "lost cause." But Mark, through perseverance and persuasion, is able to finally induce the administrators at Sloan-Kettering to admit her. The hospital, Mark has found out from his own reading and research, has the most sophisticated cancer therapy equipment on earth, and is the workplace of the cream of medicine's finest minds.

Even the machines and manpower at Sloan-Kettering, however, are not able to offer a reversal of Robin's condition. Her radiologist at Sloan-Kettering, one of the most respected masters of the profession in America, says he cannot realistically promise any longer life extension than the four to eight months the young doctor at Good Samaritan estimated. And even this life extension, he says, will only be possible with a full course of radiotherapy, followed by chemotherapy. Robin shows no reluctance to begin the radiation treatments, since the tumor in her chest is already threatening to block off her esophagus, and thus strangle her, and is also close to blocking off an artery in her neck, which will also kill her. She has great fear of the pain of chemotherapy, though, and has not decided she will undergo it.

The radiation is also painful — it is the first, Robin believes, of the treatments that will eventually transform her life into one of constant misery. She is given radiation consisting of 300 "rads" on a regular basis, which causes her to become sick at her stomach, and very weak. She can feel the rays from the cobalt radiation slowly singe the inside of her throat. Soon her throat is so badly burned that it stings almost all the time. It hurts her to swallow, but if she does not constantly wet her throat with water, she begins to feel fire in it. To eat, she must numb her throat with the topical anesthetic Xylocain, which only helps slightly.

For her last radiation treatment, she is given 3,000 "rads," ten times the amounts thus far given at any one time. As she lies there, she can feel her skin "cook" from the inside out. Two technicians are with her, one of whom tells her it is impossible for her to feel the radiation. But after that technician leaves, the other technician tells her that, yes, many patients have noticed immediate radiation burns, even while the treatment is going on. The radiation treatment only lasts for two minutes, but, to Robin, it seems like an hour.

Afterwards, she sips an icy malted milk, which is what the hospital's dietician has recommended as the best food for her, and wonders if she can endure chemotherapy when it begins. As soon as the malted is in her stomach, she feels nauseous, and as she begins to gag, she vows not to undergo chemotherapy at all, because of the constant, wretching, flu-like symptoms that it will cause.

Each day seems to bring a painful new procedure. One day the doctors have to cut slits in her feet to stick tubes into. The tubes carry a dye that makes Robin's lymphatic system visible by x-ray. The dye is also injected between her toes. Only a topical anesthetic is used, and even after the doctors are finished, her feet hurt, and walking is excruciating.

On another day, the doctors have to inject dye into her arm, so that it will travel to her kidneys and make them visible by x-rays. The doctor performing the procedure tells her that the dye will burn a little as it curculates through her vein. But the dye feels molten in her arm.

"Something is wrong," she blurts. "It hurts!"

"It's supposed to hurt," the doctor tells her.

"Not like this!" The pain in her arm is becoming unbearable. The doctor reluctantly agrees to momentarily stop the procedure. Soon her arm holds a golf-ball sized lump, proof that the dye never entered the vein. The doctor tells her he must try it in her other arm, and he inserts the needle.

"It's happening again," she pants, trying to remain calm.

"That's impossible."

But her other arm begins to swell, too. "We'll have to try again," the doctor says.

For the first time since her treatment has begun, Robin breaks down and cries in front of a doctor. "Just leave me alone; please leave me alone."

But he insists, and on the third attempt his efforts are successful. Within an hour, though, Robin's arms are so inflamed and distended that the elbow joints are no longer visible. Traces of the dye will remain in her arms for many months.

She grows even weaker as the treatment continues. She finishes the last of her 14 cobalt treatments on July 31, about two weeks after they had begun, but is unable to leave the hospital for another week. She is too weak, nauseous, swollen and burned to be sent home. She had begun vomiting very frequently after the radiation had begun, and also had developed almost constant diarrhea.

For emotional support, a psychologist and priest visit her at least once a day. In late July, the psychologist says to her, "Robin, the kids have got to know, and it would be best if it came from you."

The children wait with Mark in a downstairs chapel at Sloan-Kettering, unable to go up to their mother's floor, which is off-limits to children.

Robin takes Jimmy in first. A stoic eight-year-old, he neither cries nor asks for details. Robin does not believe that he is accepting what is happening to her.

Dora, eleven, sobs when Robin tells her she has cancer. Dora has seen two uncles, an aunt and a cousin die from cancer in the past few years. She doesn't need to be told what cancer is.

When both children go out to the car, Robin sits with Mark. "I can't leave them," she says. "Mark, find me eight years."

"I will," he says.

She doesn't believe he will be able to, and neither does he.

Mark goes to the New York Academy of Medicine and purchases time on their computer. He has worked with computers and understands their use. He begins gathering information on histiocytic lymphoma, and following it up with research in the

Academy's library. The search yields information, but no real hope. Mark finds out that the average patient with the disease lives 1.3 years, but that people with cases as advanced as Robin's generally do not live much beyond six months.

Mark scours the world's research on the disease, and finds out that Sloan-Kettering does, indeed, appear to lead Europe and the industrialized Oriental nations in treatment of the disease. Mark meets with the doctors at Sloan-Kettering, and obtains additional research materials from them. Soon he has boxes of articles and books. None of it offers hope.

During the first week of August, the widow of a former friend of Mark's calls to urge him to research naturalistic, holistic cancer therapy. Two years ago, the woman's husband, suffering from cancer, had consulted a physician who had attempted to cure the man's cancer by bolstering his immune strength with a program of health-stimulation. The man had died, but his dying had been relatively peaceful and painless, and the man's widow had become convinced that if he had tried the naturalistic approach earlier in the course of the disease, he might have survived. Like Robin, he had been pronounced terminal, and had only turned to the holistic therapy as a last resort.

Mark types "holistic cancer therapy" into the computer, and nothing comes up. He punches in "naturalistic cancer therapy," and again gets no response. Finally he keys in "unorthodox cancer therapy," and is referred to the work of Linus Pauling, Ph.D., on vitamin C and cancer, and that of Max Gerson, M.D., on holistic cancer therapy. He locates books by Dr. Gerson and Dr. Pauling that are in the Academy's library.

Both books, which advance the idea that the body's own defense system can kill cancer cells, make sense to Mark. He knows that immunotherapy — the using of pharmaceutical chemicals to bolster the body's own immunity to cancer — is highly regarded in the medical community, and thinks that this naturalistic form of immunotherapy at least deserves to be considered innocent until proven guilty. The idea that cancer can be defeated merely by stimulating a patient's health seems rather simplistic to Mark, but it seems at least worthy of investigation.

As he studies the holistic approach, he discovers that the health-stimulative programs advocated by naturalistic cancer therapists are actually quite complex. Patients, Mark finds, are advised to use everything at their disposal to try to kill their own cancer cells, including strict dietary regimens and food supplements, internal cleansing of the body, positive thinking, exercise, and various lifestyle changes, such as avoidance of cigarettes or toxic chemicals. The concept that this could make a person healthier seems reasonable to Mark — but could it cure a person of cancer?

Mark voices some questions about this approach to several doctors, but is rebuffed with responses that range from sarcastic cynicism to merely lack of interest. The doctors he talks to believe that modern, technological medicine has so distantly eclipsed naturalistic medicine that naturalistic medicine no longer has anything to offer to the modern doctor.

Mark is discouraged, because he has considerable respect for the doctors he had been consulting with and reading about. Nevertheless, they are offering him no hope, and he feels that he and Robin have, quite simply, nothing to lose by trying the naturalistic approach.

He brings her crystals of vitamin C. Dr. Pauling's book said that vitamin C not only stimulates the body's immune response, but also helps healthy cells withstand the rigors of radiation. He also begins bringing her wholesome food to eat, including organically grown oatmeal.

The nurses and the hospital dietician make light of Mark's and Robin's efforts to improve her health. To them, this couple seems to be grasping pathetically at straws. But Mark is undaunted, and begins to visit health food stores to find more books on naturalistic medicine. It is the first time in his life he has ever been inside a health food store. He reads a number of books by naturalistic doctors, and becomes more and more intrigued by the claims they make. Mark gradually abandons his research of the technological, mechanistic approach to hystiocytic lymphona. If the technological approach had offered even a shred of hope, Mark would have made time to study it. But it did not.

When Robin first reads a small book about the approach of Dr. William Donald Kelley, she throws the book across the room. "I'll *never* use this program!" she shouts at Mark.

The book she has been reading describes a challenging regimen of dietary change, internal cleansing, food supplementation and lifestyle alteration that seems all too difficult to Robin.

"They've got you doing something every ten minutes on this program! They even make you take enemas with coffee. Gross!"

Mark doesn't argue with her. If she doesn't want to do this program, he knows he can't make her.

When he comes back the next afternoon, she has retrieved the book and is reading it again. Mark volunteers to look into Dr. Kelley and the program he has devised.

Mark finds out that Dr. Kelley is an orthodontist with several other health-related degrees who at one time had a severe, presumably terminal case of cancer. Dr. Kelley, however, cured himself of the cancer through measures similar to the ones he now lectures, teaches and writes about. The measures he advocates are all common-sense health-stimulation techniques, such as nutritional therapy and internal cleansing. Dr. Kelley, Mark finds, is highly regarded by doctors who use naturalistic therapies. Many holistic physicians, Mark discovers, attend lectures and seminars given by Dr. Kelley, and discuss with him their work with patients. Dr. Kelley, an expert in the application of computers to medicine, has amassed a fund of information on health and disease in a series of computers, and he shares this information with doctors who consult with him. Some of these doctors, Mark finds out, are in the New York area.

Mark visits a young Connecticut physician recommended by a friend, who has worked with Dr. Kelley. This doctor first began to consult with Dr. Kelley while still in medical school, and has grown increasingly impressed with the wealth of information on human health and resistance to disease that Dr. Kelley has acquired. The young physician tells Mark that he will try to help Robin, if it is possible for him to do so, and will use Dr. Kelley's computerized informational services to help devise a health-stimulating program for her. Mark is dubious.

On the day Robin checks out of Sloan-Kettering, her radiologist takes Mark into a private room to talk to him.

"The preliminary tumor diminished in size quickly in response to radiation," he tells Mark, "but that means that it will probably come back quickly." He tells Mark that the tumor will probably return in three or four months, and will then be extremely hard to stop. Chemotherapy, he says, will then be needed to temporarily slow the tumor's growth.

This trip home, the radiologist says, may be Robin's last.

CHAPTER THREE

Discovery

After you lose hope, after you accustom yourself to the feeling of knowing absolutely that your death is near and cannot be stopped, you begin to avoid people who try to pry you away from your hopelessness. The slow process of losing hope is more painful than the enduring of an accepted despair, so you try not to be seduced by the glimmer of optimism that seems to come so easily to those who are not directly threatened.

In the last stages of abandoning your hope, you discover who you trust the most. The people whose encouragement and optimism you abandon last, you realize, are the ones that you have invested the most confidence in. It is sometimes surprising to learn who you really trust. Often it's not who you would think it might be. Sometimes you find yourself trusting a doctor — a stranger — more than your own husband or father, and sometimes it's just the opposite.

In any case, when you lay down your hope, you find out what you *really* believe, and who you really believe, because the time for kidding yourself is long past. You feel as if you are seeing things with crystal clarity for the first time.

Once you have accepted hopelessness as a part of your life, you drift into a strong feeling of detachment, of unreality — you seem to be outside of your own body, watching events occur with cool, unemotional eyes. You see things happen to yourself that would once have unleashed in you a torrent of feelings — fear, anger, sadness — but which now only seem . . . interesting, or unusual. This cold objectivity reinforces your feeling that you are, for the first time in your life, seeing things as they really are.

You realize, after awhile, that you have arrived at a greater understanding than ever before about life and other people. But there is only a sad feeling of irony in this realization, no joy, because you know that you are only seeing life more and more clearly because you are moving further and further away from it.

And when people try to pull you back into life, back into the pain and fear of feeling real and grasping at straws and hoping against hope, you get angry at them — or you just tell them you're tired, and you roll over, and you close your eyes until they go away.

Robin does not want to go with Mark to meet Dr. Kelley, an idea Mark had proposed as soon as she had returned home from the hospital. The trip to meet the well-known holistic doctor threatens her placid lack of positive expectation — it threatens to plunge her back into the highs and lows of hopefulness, a roller-coaster ride she no longer feels she has the strength for. Over the past few weeks, she has become familiar with hopelessness, and no longer considers inevitability a horrible thing. In a strange way, she has discovered, inevitability, even of one's own death, can create a feeling of security.

As Robin helps Mark pack her luggage for the trip, she finds herself being tugged away from hopelessness, and the feeling is painful. When she had first become sick, she remembers, she would have given anything to have had something to hope for. But now. . . .

The trip itself hurts. On the airplane, which is unusually warm as it wings west beneath a hot August sun, Robin shivers beneath three wool blankets. Her fellow passengers look at her curiously as they strip off their coats and jackets. She sips water during the entire cross-country flight, trying to quell the parched aching in her badly burned throat. She is unable to eat, because of her throat's burns and because she is still suffering from the nausea of radiation sickness.

They rent a car in Seattle and begin the five-hour drive over the Cascade Mountains to the town of Winthrop, Washington, site of the Kelley Foundation and residence of Dr. W. D. Kelley, medical computer expert and proponent of holistic health programs. Mark is amazed at the awesome mountain-pass views, but he is unable to persuade Robin, lying prone in the back seat, to raise her head and look out. Twice they have to stop the car so that she can vomit.

Mark, who prompted the trip, is far from optimistic. A pragmatic realist, he knows that the information he has thus far gathered on Dr. Kelley's work is hardly enough to inspire complete faith; he has read only one book and a few magazine articles. He has talked to people who have said complimentary things about Dr. Kelley — most notably the young Connecticut physician — but most of these people are short-term acquaintances.

No small reason for the Winthrop visit is Mark's determination to meet Dr. Kelley and measure the man himself. The Connecticut doctor has told Mark that a personal visit to Dr. Kelley's home town is not necessary for people who wish to employ Dr. Kelley's ideas. A personal talk with Dr. Kelley is always instructive, the doctor has told Mark, but the program can be easily administered without it. But Mark, who is no gambler, feels that they must make the trip and meet the man before they adopt his ideas.

"I think somebody has played a bad joke on us," says Robin as she slumps back in the seat of the car. They are parked before the Kelley Foundation, which has turned out to be nothing more than a sheet-metal roofed, two-bedroom house in a modest Winthrop residential neighborhood. Mark is equally underwhelmed by the splendor, or lack thereof, of the Kelley Foundation, an association he had hoped would be housed in a facility not unlike those composing Sloan-Kettering: one that is sleek, electronic, modern — *confidence-inspiring.* Mark considers turning the car around and avoiding a night in rural Washington.

But as Mark glumly ponders the situation, a woman bounds out the door of the house and effusively greets Mark and Robin. She explains that she is a recovered cancer patient, one who "owes my life" to Dr. Kelley. Six years ago, she says, she was pronounced terminal by doctors at an East Coast hospital, but contradicted their pronouncement by recovering under the care of a doctor who was working with Dr. Kelley. Her doctor, she says, using information from Dr. Kelley's computer bank, created a health-stimulating program for her that caused her immune mechanisms to defeat her cancer. The woman, a glowing magnet of enthusiasm and energy, makes Dr. Kelley sound heroic.

Mark thinks to himself that either this Dr. Kelley is really onto something, or he is clever enough to hire good actors to represent him. Either possibility, thinks Mark, ever the skeptic, is quite feasible.

And then Dr. Kelley himself comes out, and stops briefly on the way to his car. In his late '40s or early '50s, sandy-haired, casually dressed, he gives no impression, as he introduces himself with a slight Kansas drawl, of being a computer wizard or a medical pioneer. Mark, accustomed to the more high-powered presentations favored by the Sloan-Kettering medical technocrats, is not terribly impressed. Robin, however, likes the carefully gentle manner of the doctor. The woman who had recovered from cancer puts her arm around Dr. Kelley's shoulders and says, "You don't know how lucky you are to have found this man." Dr. Kelley looks genuinely embarrassed, tugs himself away, and slides into his car.

The next day Dr. Kelley spends all morning with Mark and Robin. He explains the approach he has developed and tells Robin that her program will not be easy. He tells her that she is as sick as anyone he has ever tried to help. He tells Mark that, as Robin's husband and helper, he will have to spend long hours taking care of her, and that they will probably have to spend hundreds of dollars on wholesome food products and nutritional supplements. However, Robin notices, in Dr. Kelley's assessments of all the negative aspects of the recovery program, he never seems to assume that hers is a hopeless case. He talks as if whether or not she will recover depends largely upon her own actions, rather than upon the dictums of current survival statistics or upon the state of the medical arts. Robin is not used to relating to her disease in any but a passive manner, and she finds it strangely disquieting to think about *fighting* the cancer, as she would fight a head cold or a case of heartburn.

For a few moments, when she becomes swept up with the idea of being able to conspire against the cancer, and battle it, and defeat it, she finds that her detachment has dissolved, and that she feels once again as if she is the inhabitant of her body, and not a stranger standing outside it. But then the fear returns, and the sadness, and she regrets her momentary burst of confidence.

For several days they stay in Winthrop, which has turned out to be an idyllic mountain village, pristine and immaculate, and consult with Dr. Kelley. After the first talk, Dr. Kelley invites Mark to come back in the afternoon if he has any more questions. Mark returns with two pages of questions that day, and three the next morning, and four pages more the morning after that.

As he continues his discussions with Dr. Kelley, Mark conducts a personal fact-finding mission on the doctor, researching him as intensely as he had researched hystiocytic lymphona on the Med-Line computer. He talks to many of the people in Winthrop who know the doctor, and with all the medical people who come to Dr. Kelley's office to talk with him. Mark even checks with the county assessor's office to see what property Dr. Kelley owns, and finds that the doctor owns a 160-acre farm outside town, where he is conducting an extensive research project on preserving nutrients in stored foods. Mark is impressed with the farm project, because it indicates to him that Dr. Kelley has made a long-term investment in his town and in his field of work.

Mark and Robin are told by Dr. Kelley, who has degrees in dentistry, orthodontics, biology and chemistry, about how he once was told he had a terminal case of cancer. In the mid-1960s, Dr. Kelley's internist had told him that he would die within a matter of weeks from a metasticized pancreatic cancer, one of the deadliest forms of the disease. Dr. Kelley, who by that time had an extensive background in nutrition and biochemistry, embarked upon a self-created course of nutritional therapy, exercise, lifestyle change, and positive thinking, and began to feel better. Dr. Kelley had hoped to improve his quality of life, but had not expected to extend his life with this program, so he was as surprised as his internist when he passed the date of his presumed death. Encouraged, he refined his program, and began talking large doses of food supplements and engaging in internal cleansing procedures. Soon, he was spending almost the entire day trying to stimulate his own health. As he gradually recovered, he knew that he had stumbled across a remarkable scientific lesson, and began strenuously researching naturalistic medical practices. He found that only a modest body of literature existed on naturalistic medicine, and particularly naturalistic cancer therapy, so he began programming his own office's computer with all the information he could find that related to immune stimulation. By the late 1960s, he had amassed a considerable body of information in his computer system, which he had expanded, and he began working as a consultant to physicians who used whole-systems, metabolic therapies for the treatment of degenerative diseases, such as cancer, cardiovascular disease, diabetes, and arthritis. The physicians Doctor Kelley began working with started to unofficially refer to themselves as "metabolic doctors."

It became Dr. Kelley's contention that most diseases could be defeated if the body's metabolism was powerfully stimulated with an immune-enhancing program of dietary change, food supplementation, structural and emotional therapies, internal cleansing, and lifestyle change. He had also come to believe that each person required a unique, fully individualized program, one tailored to each person's specific needs, and he had learned how to use his computers to help doctors provide these programs for patients. Thousands of patients, by the late 1970s, had benefited greatly from the information provided by Dr. Kelley and the metabolic physicians. Many of the patients had been gravely ill. Some had been as ill as Robin Fonwood.

Mark and Robin sit in the high grass at the end of a gravel road on the top of a mountain. They have come up here on their way out of town. Robin, who has begun a temporary, modified version of her program, feels somewhat better. Her throat is not as sore and she is not so nauseous.

The wind-bent grass, dry as straw in the late-summer heat, whispers noisily as they stare across the valley. "When we left today," says Robin, "Dr. Kelley took me aside and told me I better work hard. I think he's worried that I'm going to ruin his reputation."

It is the first time in weeks that Mark has heard her joke. Mark, very pleased, tries to joke back, but finds he can't.

"Do you really think doing all those . . . things . . . will help?" asks a middle-aged friend of Mark's mother. "Shouldn't you do what your *doctor* says?"

Robin, a guest in her mother-in-law's home in Florida, where they have come for a visit after leaving Washington, reminds the woman that the program she is on *was* devised by her doctor.

"Well," says the woman, "I guess it's your life."

Robin and Mark have become accustomed to the skepticism of family and friends about her program; they are patient with the attitude because they until recently shared it. Robin's doubts about the benefits of her program, devised by her Connecticut physician with the help of Dr. Kelley, have faded away as she has begun to feel better. Mark's dubiousness has been overcome by the long hours of study he has done on naturalistic medicine.

Robin has much less nausea now, a week after leaving Washington, and her throat feels almost normal. She has more energy and appetite than at any time since she began radiotherapy. Her adjustment to the program devised for her has been relatively easy, simply because she feels noticeably better when she engages in the recommended procedures. She had, for example, a strong distaste for the idea of taking enemas with coffee when she had first heard about the program, but now does not mind taking them at all, because they markedly decrease her nausea. Dr. Kelley had explained to her that caffeine from coffee, when taken in a retention enema, enters the liver directly through the colon's portal vein, and stimulates that organ to excrete toxic substances into the bile system. The periodic build-up in her liver of these toxic materials, Robin has discovered, accounts largely for her nausea. Now when she begins to feel sick at her stomach, she merely takes a brief coffee enema, and the nausea virtually always abates.

Similarly, taking dozens of food supplements every day, which once had seemed to her a significant annoyance, now is almost a pleasure, since the influx of nutrients in the supplements often seems to bring her increased feelings of strength and well-being.

As she and Mark work on her program, she learns more than she ever has about her body and its health. She learns that her energy levels and sensitivity to pain and emotional upset can be regulated through certain dietary practices. She learns, for example, that high amounts of calcium and magnesium can calm her nerves and put her to sleep, even when she is nervous or in pain, and that certain fruits and juices can shift her body's acid-alkaline balance, which can strongly affect her emotional outlook. She learns that her liver, which she had never thought about before starting the program, is a collecting pool for toxic materials, but that she can excrete these materials through a mild, naturalistic procedure called a "liver flush." She finds out that she feels inordinately better after one of these "liver flushes." She finds that many of her aches and pains can be alleviated by a visit to a chiropractor — a type of health professional she would never have considered visiting in the past. She learns that she has difficulty expressing negative feelings, and, on the advice of her Connecticut doctor, she begins to learn techniques that drain off anger and fear. These techniques leave her feeling more relaxed and calm than she has felt since she became ill. She finds that if she avoids sugary foods, she has fewer physical and emotional highs-and-lows, and feels more in control of her physical and emotional condition. She finds that if she makes herself take a nap every day, whether she feels like it or not, that she feels better the entire rest of the day.

The longer she stays with the program, the more she realizes that she has, as she has grown older, gradually gotten away from taking good care of herself. She begins to appreciate how completely she has gotten out of the habit of fulfilling her own needs as they have arisen. She has become adept, she realizes, at taking care of Jimmy and Dora and Mark and Marie and her mother . . . just about everyone, in fact — except herself.

One evening, sitting alone in a quiet bedroom, she experiences a sudden flash of certainty. It is time, she realizes, for her to realign the balance of her life. The time has passed for her to be always telling people not to bother about getting her what she needs, whether it is a handful of vitamins or some fresh-squeezed juice. She speaks her thoughts out loud, quietly, but with absolute sureness: "I *deserve* to be cared for." From that moment on, she realizes, things will be different. She knows that she might recover, or that she might not, but no matter what happens, she knows she will no longer feel guilty about what has happened to her, or about anything she has said or done. And she will no longer worry about how well or how badly she will react to having cancer.

When she stops worrying about how she will react to the possibly painful future, she loses much of her fear of that future. When she realizes that she doesn't have to be a hero, she feels much more free than she has felt since the first x-rays.

That night she sleeps well, and the next morning she tells Mark to have the kids flown down — together they will all go to Disney World in Orlando.

For two days they tour Disney World. Robin even leaves her wheelchair to go on some of the rides. For two days, life seems normal. Robin forgets that she is going to die.

The doctor is livid. "I don't care if ten doctors in Connecticut think that it's a well-constructed program," he tells Mark and Robin. "I say it's quackery!"

The young doctor, the one who had first discovered Robin's cancer, has heard of programs like the one Robin is on and thinks they are of no benefit. He is insisting that Robin begin a course of chemotherapy.

"But we've talked to half a dozen people that have been really helped by this kind of program," says Mark, who is holding onto his temper. "We just talked to a businessman in Florida whose wife was saved by it. She's supposed to be dead now, and she's playing eighteen holes of golf every day."

"There are always a certain percent of spontaneous remissions," says the doctor. "And did you see this woman's medical records? Are you certain she ever even had cancer? I'll tell you one thing," says the doctor. "No amount of vitamins and enemas is ever going to cure cancer! Modern medicine left that kind of stuff behind so long ago that it isn't even funny."

Mark suddenly realizes that in the past eight weeks he has learned more about naturalistic medicine and nutrition than this doctor now knows. "Well, doctor," Mark says quietly, "it's Robin's decision, and I agree with her — she's going to try this program out, and if it doesn't work, then we'll talk about chemotherapy."

The doctor drops the folder in his hands so that he can point his finger at Mark. "If you put off this chemotherapy," the doctor says, "you're killing her. You'll be responsible for her death."

Mark nods, and they get up to leave. On the way out the door, Robin gives Mark a big smile, a very strong smile, for which he is very grateful.

CHAPTER FOUR

The New Approach To Cancer

When you first begin to feel that you are regaining control of a life gone chaotic with illness, you feel like a child at Christmas. Nothing could be more wonderful, you think, than merely commanding the course of your own life. After a long period of feeling helpless and passive, hostage to a disease you believed was far more powerful than yourself, even the slightest exercise of personal power feels extraordinary. If, for example, you have felt sick at your stomach for months, and you finally learn how to eliminate this nausea, you feel as if you have become the most powerful person on earth.

If the disease you are learning to dominate is cancer, you feel a special pride, a unique sense of potency. Cancer, you know, is a disease that people surrender to. When people learn they have cancer, they either give up and die, or they hand over their lives to doctors, obeying with almost child-like obedience every dictum of their physicians, even if these doctors' proposals contradict what they want for their own lives. When you begin to overpower your cancer, you feel singularly independent, like a commanding general.

You know that you may still die of cancer, because the disease is tenacious. Maybe it will never go into remission. Maybe it will go away, and then come back. You know that the cancer may lie dormant for five years, or fifteen years, and then strike you down suddenly, before you have adequate time to again marshall your resources. You know that cancer occurs in recovered cancer patients much more often than it does in people who have never had the disease — particularly if the patient has undergone a therapy like radiation, which mutates cells and causes long-delayed cancer.

But after you have experienced that first surge of powerfulness, your fears about the future are never again so fierce.

You no longer lie trembling in bed, like a child listening for monsters outside the window, wondering what this awful disease will do to you next. You no longer feel like a leaf in the wind, blown helplessly about by circumstances beyond your control. Cancer may win the fight, or you may win the fight . . . but there *will* be a fight.

And with your new sense of yourself comes a question, one you can't escape: Why wasn't I like this before? If you had been like this, you think, you might not have come down with cancer in the first place. If you hadn't "burned the candle at both ends," and been careless about your health, and indulged in unimportant pleasures like junk food and cigarettes, which seemed so irresistible before you learned the true limit of your will-power, maybe you could have avoided your problem before it was a problem. If you had, over the past few years, been more concerned about your own well-being, and not put everyone else in the family first, maybe your immune system would have had the strength to resist the microscopic malignancies that grew unchallenged, and then threatened to kill you.

You realize that you are now totally aware of the changes your body goes through, changes that would once have escaped your notice.

If you had previously been so aware of the subtle shifts the body experiences on its way from health to sickness, you might have been able to keep your cancer from developing. You can become immersed in regret about having allowed your cancer to develop.

But one morning you wake up and realize that this haunting remorse has itself become destructive to your health. So you decide to answer, once and for all, the question: "Why wasn't I like this before?" And you find the answer is obvious: "I wasn't like this because I hadn't learned the things cancer has taught me."

Realizing this, you stop regretting that you have cancer. And then you are stronger than you have ever before been, and you know will be strong until you die.

Robin, back home in Long Island, fights her cancer every day, and becomes increasingly sure that she has no small voice in the matter of whether or not she will continue to live. She also becomes deeply convinced that she will be able to control the manner of her death, if death is unavoidable. She is virtually certain that, even if her tumors become so large that they inhibit the function of a vital organ — and thus kill her — she will nonetheless be able to avoid many of the metabolic disruptions commonly associated with cancer. She has learned to have little fear of cachexia, or gradual wasting away due to lack of nourishment, the side-effect that had turned her brother, like so many other cancer patients, into a pitiful human skeleton. Cachexia, she has come to believe, can be overcome with a careful nutritional program. She has learned to quell her nausea, and has regained much of her strength and stamina. She no longer has nightmares about succumbing to some of the ghastly symptoms suffered by patients she had known at Sloan-Kettering, such as vomiting diarrhea, or going blind, or being covered with open sores. Her Connecticut physician, with whom she talks almost every day, has told her that cancer patients on strenuous health-stimulating programs have a much greater resistance to cancer-associated debilitating symptoms than patients who are careless about supporting their systems.

With Mark's help, Robin spends almost all day, every day, trying to regain her health. She juices quarts of fresh, organic fruits and vegetables every morning, prepares her meals with exacting care, takes several coffee enemas every day, does periodic liver flushes and mild purges of her gastrointestinal tract, visits her chiropractor and emotional counselor, does light exercise, takes naps, and each day takes dozens of food supplements.

During the early autumn, she feels much better; she experiences the first flush of power over her situation. The feeling is exhilarating, and boosts her confidence greatly. In late autumn, though, she begins to feel much worse. She becomes bedridden, depressed and feverish. Her Connecticut doctor tells her that this is actually a good sign, a signal that her body is killing malignant cells and flushing them into her eliminative systems. She is feeling ill, he tells her, because these dead cancer cells are stressing her organs of elimination. She must be careful, he says, to avoid engaging in immune-stimulating procedures so vigorously that she severely over-burdens these sensitive organs, because doing so could cause her to die.

Feeling as badly as she does, however, she wonders if he is just pacifying her. Maybe she is dying, she thinks. The idea frightens her, but it doesn't terrify her, as it had last summer. If she does die, she thinks, hers will not be a painful, pathetic, ghoulish death, and it will be a death that she will fight every step of the way.

She struggles harder than ever. Mark is on the phone every day with her Connecticut doctor, who is in almost constant contact with Dr. Kelley. One month Mark's telephone bill is $1,600.

At night now, she sometimes stops breathing. Mark must sit beside her as she sleeps, listening for her breath. Every night for over two weeks she periodically takes a deep breath, then issues a long sigh, then . . . nothing. Mark has to smack her back to make her breathe again. The condition is unnerving for both of them, and exhausting for Mark.

One night, as she is preparing for bed, she takes a pharmaceutical drug prescribed for a localized infection she has developed. As soon as she swallows the drug, she goes into anaphylactic shock. Her tongue swells up so quickly that she is barely able to tell Mark what has happened before she loses her ability to speak. She slumps onto her bed and begins to turn blue. Mark springs for the phone and calls her doctor in Connecticut. He says there is not enough time to get her to the hospital; she will strangle if Mark doesn't act instantly. He tells Mark to pour an Epsom Salts solution into her throat, and give her an immediate Epsom Salts enema. When the Epsom Salts' magnesium touches her tongue and enters her system, relaxing her smooth muscle tissue, the swelling subsides as rapidly as it had begun. Robin, jolted by her narrow escape from death, stays up and talks with Mark for several hours before she is able to fall asleep.

As winter comes, Robin continues to feel physically ill, but mentally resolute. As late December approaches, though, Robin and Mark begin to get edgy. The date will soon arrive that is Robin's "scheduled" time of death. Without chemotherapy, none of her doctors had expected her to last more than four or five months past August. Mark remembers the warning the radiologist had given him when they left Sloan-Kettering in August: "the tumor will probably return in three or four months, and will then be extremely hard to stop."

As Christmas approaches, Robin's stamina vanishes, and it gets harder and harder for her to breathe.

"You played around with that program too long, Mark, and now it's time to pay the price." Robin's young Long Island doctor, still angry at Mark and Robin for delaying her chemotherapy, fixes Mark with a glare. "The extreme shortness of breath she is now experiencing is almost certainly a sign that the primary tumor is again pressing against her trachea. It will be very difficult to slow the tumor growth this time. I'm afraid that she won't live more than six to eight days. We'll give her oxygen when it gets really bad, but that won't be enough."

"I came to arrange for x-rays," says Mark. "Shouldn't we make sure there is a tumor pressing against her windpipe before we start the chemo?"

"I don't know what else it could possibly be, Mark. With your permission, I'll schedule her for chemotherapy in the morning."

"Maybe it's just scarring of her lungs from the radiation treatments. The radiologist said that scarring of her lungs might cause shortness of breath. Maybe that's all this is."

The physician becomes exasperated with Mark for "playing doctor." "I don't think it's radiation fibrosis, Mark. I do think I should discuss this directly with Robin," he says.

"She doesn't feel well enough to come in," Mark says, "and she's having a real hard time talking over the phone, because of her breathing." Mark stands up. "Please just schedule the x-rays."

The doctor also stands up. The two men, wills implacable, face each other, both knowing they are on a collision course. "I can't be responsible for any delays in her treatment," says the doctor. "Not if she's my patient."

"That's your choice, doctor." Mark is gone.

Mark holds Robin's arm as she slowly walks to the car. They are on their way to Connecticut for x-rays. She sits up in the front seat as they drive, but can only respond in short, breathy phrases to his conversaiton. Her breath comes in a long, slow wheeze.

But if she is frightened, she doesn't show it. Mark is proud of her spirit now, a defiant spirit that stands in stark contrast to the "whipped pup" attitude she had had while still a patient at Sloan-Kettering. He has never admired her more, and feels as if he is learning many things from her about positive thinking. From the way she idly smiles at the frosty Christmas-time scenery, he thinks that she is totally confident that she is recovering. He does not know that she wrote a letter to Dora and Jimmy before they had left, telling them goodbye, and that her smile comes from a peacefulness that exists independently of her hopes for a long life.

The physician they are going to visit, who has agreed to perform the diagnostic x-rays at the request of Robin's Connecticut doctor, leaves them alone for almost an hour while he studies the x-rays. Each minute that ticks away hurts them, because they have learned that good medical news tends to come quickly, while bad news — generally not issued without the certainty of corroboration and cross-checking — arrives more slowly. They fear that this doctor, unfamiliar with Robin's case, is consulting with his colleagues, trying to think of a gentle way to tell this woman that she not only has cancer, but is in a situation so grave that she might not live a week.

When the doctor finally returns to the small visitation room that Mark and Robin have been waiting in, one hour and twenty minutes after he had left them, his face is grey with concern. As she notes his expression, Robin, who has become an expert at "reading" doctors and nurses, begins to once again feel that strange feeling of floating outside of her own body, of being able to watch things happen from above. A terrible thing is about to befall her, she thinks, and she doesn't want to feel it.

"I have something very difficult to tell you," the doctor begins — and Mark can feel his feet go cold — "so I won't beat around the bush. You've lost about 90 percent of the function of your left lung because of fibrosis. It's a very severe case. If you . . ."

"But what about the tumor?" Mark interrupts.

"What tumor?"

"The tumor right in here," Robin says, touching her chest.

"There isn't any tumor there. There isn't any sign of cancer anywhere. Did you think there still was?"

Neither Mark nor Robin answer him because they are holding each other and jumping up and down and crying and shouting, which Robin should not be physically capable of doing, but which she is.

They call Robin's Connecticut doctor, who is ecstatic at the news, then drive straight home. All the way home, relief washes over Robin like warm water, soothing fears and worries that she hadn't even known she had. She keeps telling herself "it isn't over yet," but in her heart she knows it is. She knows that she is in command of the situation, and that she will allow nothing to stop her total recovery. Her Connecticut doctor has already told her about deep-breathing exercises that will begin to restore the function of her lung, and she practices them on the way home.

When they get home, they go next door to Robin's house, where the kids are, and soon everyone is awake and every light in the house is on. Both families are so jubilant that Mark has to shout into the phone to be heard as he calls Robin's parents, and his parents, and other family members, and close friends.

The next morning, a Saturday, Mark and Robin send the kids to Marie's house, and they go Christmas shopping, alone. Robin must walk very slowly, and must often stop and sit down. As noon approaches, soft crystals of snow sift down from the sky, whitewashing everything that is not already luminous and clean. Robin and Mark shuffle past department store windows — each of which promises a happy holiday — neither of them caring if they buy anything, both of them feeling as if they are very young again, and have just met each other, and have no problems, and never will have any problems that they can't solve. They speak infrequently, as peaceful people sometimes do.

After awhile, they stop talking altogether, content to just hold hands, walk slowly, feel the snow come down and look into windows bright with color and hot lights and the promise of happiness to come.

PART TWO

Cancer Can Be Understood

At every crossing on the road that leads to the future, each progressive spirit is opposed by a thousand men appointed to guard the past.

—Maurice Maeterlinck

CHAPTER FIVE

The Foundations of Metabolic Therapy

Nothing so delights the members of the medical profession as much as the concept of a "breakthrough." Virtually every fresh season brings some "new medical discovery," one heralded with a ceremonious pomp rivaling that of a debutante's coming-out party. Only makers of soap flakes and instant pudding match medical scientists in their ability to regularly produce a "new, improved" version of the product of their profession. About twenty years ago the season's sensations were the dubious introductions of tranquilizers and "pep pills," which were followed by the fad of heart transplants, then fertility drugs, and, most lately, the advent of Interferon, the "magical" anti-cancer agent that is almost certain to prove disappointing. The conventional wisdom dominating the medical profession during this century has been that if medicines keep getting stronger and healing machines keep getting bigger, then health for our nation will surely be waiting just around the corner. What nonsense!

It is highly doubtful that any disease epidemic, certainly including our current horrendous cancer epidemic, has ever been, or ever will be, solved by bombardment with medicines, machines and money. Medicines, machines and money can blunt the blow of medical crisis, but only personal, human life-changing can consistently reverse the course of epidemic disease patterns. The contagious disease epidemics of the early 1900s were ended, medical researchers have proven, by societal improvements in nutrition, sanitation, housing and hygiene, rather than by drugs or vaccines.[1] If our cancer epidemic is ever to be stemmed, it will be through similar changes. It will be through the clinical application of nutrition, internal cleansing, stress reduction and lifestyle changes—in other words, through application of naturalistic, health-building programs. Health-building programs for cancer, which stimulate the body's own immune, recuperative response to malignancy, are not "new-improved-breakthrough-discoveries." How could anyone claim that eating properly, or getting rest and exercise, are "new" ideas? These regimens, rather, are founded in the oldest tradition in healing. They come from an intellectual base that pre-dates the modern medical philosophy, which says that health can be forced into people with medicines and machines.

This approach is medicine's oldest school of thought.

The Old School

"Vitalism" is the oldest doctrine of healing. Vitalism, as defined by anthropologist Richard Grossinger, states that life "possesses properties in some manner above and beyond its physics and chemistry."[2] The vitalistic healing tradition holds that health cannot be imposed upon a living organism, but can be achieved only when that organism lives in accord with the natural laws that govern all living things. Vitalism agrees with the idea that a sum is greater than its parts, and that there will probably always be mysteries in living creatures. Because there is a respect for the unknown in this philosophy, the doctrine is part of the "pragmatic" healing approach, which says that techniques which seem to work are good techniques, even if the reasons for their success are unclear.[3] The healing power of the mind, for example, is apparent, but is mysterious. The vitalistic healing tradition is, therefore, an "empirical" science, meaning that its techniques are derived through observation of results, rather than through application of fixed principles. Because of this approach's respect for the sometimes mysterious functions of the human body, and because of its acceptance of numerous techniques that appear to be valuable, although they are not totally understandable, the vitalistic medical approach is generally characterized by use of a wide variety of natural, "non-invasive" healing techniques.

The vitalistic tradition is considered healing's oldest doctrine because it was at the heart of all ancient medicines, including those of the Chinese and Egyptians.[4] The Chinese have shown a profound respect for the human body and its recuperative powers since almost 3,000 B.C. They have been in general opposition to surgery for thousands of years, because of its invasion of the human body, which they believed could usually heal itself.[5] The Egyptians were noted for their use of an assortment of natural healing techniques, including herbology, nutrition and hygiene.[6]

In 400 B.C., Hippocrates, the "Father of Modern Medicine," formalized the vitalistic concept. He wrote what had been believed by many societies for literally thousands of years—that disease is a multifaceted, sometimes enigmatic occurrence, taking place in a complex, often puzzling world. He said that to overcome disease, which he saw as part of the natural, rhythmical rise and fall of life's energy, a person should strive to obey what seem to be the laws that govern nature. Symptoms, he felt, were signs of healing, and should be stimulated rather than suppressed. Hippocrates, who stressed the idea of balance, was basically conservative in his use of healing techniques. It was better to do nothing, he felt, than to do the wrong thing.[7]

The Hippocratic teachings are the philosophical basis of metabolic therapy, which can best be described as a therapy that seeks to improve the function of the body's entire energy exchange with the environment, or its "metabolism." Vitalistic, multi-faceted programs stimulate natural recuperation. Doctors are not always aware of every single biochemical exchange that takes place during a metabolic healing process, so they strive to give the body as much balance and support as they possibly can, so that the body can perform its own astounding recuperative feats.

Medicine As Mechanics

Shortly after the time of Hippocrates, another philosophy of healing was constructed. This school, the "mechanistic" mode of healing, currently predominates in our medical profession.[8] The mechanistic philosophy holds that all living things are essentially complex biological "machines," and can be reduced to a collection of more-or-less interchangeable, replaceable parts. This philosophy declares that fixed laws govern every aspect of biology, that all parts of all of these laws can be learned, and that correct application of these laws to a living organism can "repair" the organism of any possible malfunction. This philosophy, then, is "rational," or based upon application of set principles, rather than empirical.

The mechanistic philosophy was originated by a group of Greek physicians known as the Cnidians.[9] It was brought to its fruition, though, by the Greek physician Galen in the second century A.D. Galen forged the intellectual framework upon which rests today's most common cancer therapies—chemotherapy, surgery and radiation, which attempt to oppose symptoms and impose healing from outside the body. Galen said that medicine should be based on mechanical laws of anatomy, logic and physiology. He felt that a few major organs, including the heart, lungs and liver, were the body's primary sources of life-maintenance, rather than that proper function of all parts of the body, working as a whole, was necessary for a healthy life. Galen strongly advocated creating a special societal role for healers.[10] The Romans quickly adopted Galen's views, which meshed quite well with their attempts to compartmentalize and stratify law, government and language. In the Roman empire, the concepts of "legal" and "illegal" medicines were born.[11]

Middle Age Medicine

In the Middle Ages, the vitalistic and mechanistic modes warred for acceptance in the minds of medical practitioners. The greatest medical practitioner of the era, the Swiss physician Paracelsus, practiced a form of vitalistic medicine that incorporated the techniques of the Chinese, Egyptians and Greeks, as well as Europe's folk healers.[12] Paracelsus, who lived in the 1500s, believed that healing could best be accomplished by focusing natural healing forces, including the patient's own mind, on the disease.

The philosopher Rene Descartes greatly forwarded the mechanistic approach in the 1600s by implementing his "deductive" method of thinking into medicine.[13] The deductive method of attaining knowledge—which is done by reducing matters to their smallest, simplest components—has become not only the operant mode in medicine, but is the basis for the "scientific method" of reasoning.

New knowledge unearthed during this Renaissance era, including Harvey's discovery that the blood circulates, Koch's discovery of bacteria, and Semmelweis' discovery of the value of cleanliness during surgery, also boosted the mechanical school of medical thought. Subsequent discoveries, occurring in the Industrial Revolution of the 1800s, further enhanced mechanistic healing. These included the inventions of the x-ray, anesthetic, the hypodermic needle and antiseptic solution.

During this era, the role of the doctor became gradually more socially and economically elevated. By the 1800s, physicians had come to be regarded as advanced healing scientists, even though many of their therapies, including blood-letting and the indiscriminate use of the toxic substance mercury, were barbaric.[14] As American doctors entered the twentieth century, they had the political skill to legislate into the country's legal codes a concept that has insured the power of healers, witch doctors and barber-surgeons throughout history: the concept that a society's healer has a special link to life-saving knowledge, if not indeed to God Himself, and should thus be allowed to perform, once a member of the profession, virtually any act of his choosing, as long as it is done in the name of healing.

The Forces Shaping Modern Medicine

In America in the 1900s, medicine reached what until recently appeared to be an almost indissoluble union with technology. The marriage was consummated in 1910 with the issuing of the "Flexner Report," a powerful proclamation sponsored jointly by the newborn American Medical Association and the Carnegie Foundation, which called for almost sole reliance upon drugs and surgery as the proper tools of medicine.[15] Medical schools that adopted the precepts of the report were given windfall grants by the Carnegie Foundation. In that somewhat less cynical era, few people thought to question the fact that the Carnegie family was deeply imbedded in the young pharmaceutical drug industry.[16]

Drug companies, including those controlled by the Carnegies, began dumping dollars into medical education at an unprecedented clip. Single companies poured, by themselves, hundreds of millions of dollars into medical schools.[17] Medical students were taught that symptom-opposing procedures using drugs and surgery were easy to implement, needed virtually no cooperation from or effort by the patient, were easy to categorize and quantify, and were lucrative.

Mechanistic healing still had a strong rival in the vitalistic school, however. In the early 1900s this method of healing flourished. Samuel Hahnemann's "homeopathy," a healing technique based on stimulating symptoms, was in wide use prior to World War II, and was considered the most potent threat to mechanistic medicine. Chiropractic and osteopathy, two "structural" therapies which deal with bones and nerves, had many adherents in the early 1900s. Probably the most sophisticated of the vitalistic healers, though, were the "eclectic physicians" of the pre-World War II period. These medical doctors used the pragmatic approach of applying whatever appeared to work, even if the mechanism of action of the therapy was partly or largely mysterious. The eclectic physicians employed the techniques of folk healers, herbologists, nutritionists, hygienists, psychologists, surgeons, homeopathists, structural therapists, spiritualists and exercise therapists.[18] If there is a group that patients benefiting from metabolic anticancer programs owe a debt of gratitude to, it is that of the eclectic physicians, who were the most apparent forerunners of modern holistic health.

After World War II, with America embarked upon a course of supra-industrialism, mechanical medicine reached a zenith of predominance. For two decades after the war, anything other than mechanically-oriented medicine was sneered at as ludicrous quackery.

A rapid decline in the number of solo practitioners and a sharp increase in machine-based therapy has characterized this most recent era. People are now most commonly treated by a series of specialists, each expert in only one realm of physiology, which carries Galen's dictums on separate organ function to a logically illogical resolution.

The trend toward technological medicine has also been undeniably profitable for those in the health profession. Specialists receive more money than practitioners of general medicine, an average of at least $25,000 more per year.[19] Surgeries have become such a big business that one critic of the medical establishment, Robert Mendelsohn, M.D., estimates that approximately 2.4 million unnecessary operations, costing $4 billion, are performed each year.[20] Expenditures on technology-based medicine have risen dramatically as a percentage of the average person's income. The average family now spends over 12 per cent of its earnings on health care. The nation's financial outlay on health has increased by a factor of almost twenty since just 1950.[21]

Great sums of money have been earned by a group of industries indirectly involved in America's "health care system," which is, quite apparently, a pleasant euphemism for what is obviously a sickness care system. This group includes owners of nursing homes, makers of technological apparati, pharmaceutical companies, and health insurance firms. Makers of equipment and supplies, for example, saw an increase in their business from $3.8 million in 1950 to $300 million in 1970.[22] The number of Americans holding health insurance policies increased from somewhat more than 10 per cent of the population in 1940 to over 90 per cent today.

The pharmaceutical industry has shown the most spectacular growth. Antibiotics in the 1940s, tranquilizers in the 1950s, and birth control pills in the 1960s all helped the industry account for its current take of 12 per cent of every dollar spent in America on health.[23] The industry now generates $20 billion yearly in sales and $2 billion in profits. Drug prices have sometimes increased as much as 25 per cent per year. Drug companies are, to a large extent, non-competitive; of 51 chemical entities comprising two-thirds of all prescription drug sales, 27 have only one producer, eight have only two producers, and none have more than seven producers.[24] Drug company profits, over the past 15 years, have outranked those of all other manufacturing industries listed in the Stock Exchange.

With this economic surge in medical care has come undeniable political power. Medical lobbyists are among the best-financed and most influential in all of government, and the key executives from the health industry regularly fill the posts of the health-regulating agencies, such as the Food and Drug Administration and the National Institutes of Health. Private groups that favor the surgical-pharmaceutical approach, such as the American Medical Association and the American Cancer Society, are closely allied with health-industry corporations, and also have immense power over the federal health bureaucracy.

The societal role of the medical doctor has risen with the ascendance of the technological approach. Medical doctors are currently almost unparalleled in social, economic and intellectual influence.

With an array of forces like these lined up against natural, vitalistic medicine, it is a wonder that this tradition has been able to survive. Vitalistic medicine, though, instead of withering, has blossomed over the past two decades. Now known as "holistic health," the approach is stronger than ever. A blithe acceptance of every facet of runaway technology is no longer so rampant in our culture. We have realized in the past twenty years that machines and money cannot solve all of our problems, and that the questioning of authorities and the relying upon our own judgment not only make good sense, but are sometimes even necessary for survival.

Even during vitalistic medicine's less popular eras, however, the pioneers in the natural healing profession were extremely active. These pioneers included those involved with cancer. When public awareness of naturalistic, vitalistic healing modalities began recently to increase, an array of natural cancer therapies was awaiting inspection.

Holistic Cancer Therapy

The first Neanderthal man who had a malignant growth, decided to lie down and rest until he felt better, then eventually recovered, was the first person to recover with a "holistic cancer therapy." In all probability, every person who has ever lived has had many instances of abnormal cellular growth, which his or her body recognized, isolated, deactivated and eliminated. Thus, we all have likely been beneficiaries of "holistic cancer therapy."

The institutionalization of using the immune response to defeat malignancy is a relatively recent phenomenon, however. Only in the past decade has this endeavor been endorsed by a significant number of members of the medical community. In the late 1970s, Dr. Frank Rauscher, former head of the National Cancer Institute, set the tone for the 1980s when he said, "Immunotherapy represents the future of cancer therapy."[25]

Naturalistic, vitalistic cancer therapy has been involved in the same struggle for acceptance that all vitalistic approaches have been forced to endure. The history of medicine is grimly speckled with the systematic denigration of men of high integrity, learning and compassion who advocated and practiced naturalistic cancer therapies.

The 19th century is replete with medical pioneers who built the foundation of naturalistic cancer therapy. Nat Morris, in the *Cancer Blackout,* details the history of early naturalistic cancer therapists. One of the first, says Morris, was William Lambe, M.D., of London, who in 1809 published a paper advocating the use of nutritional therapy for patients.[26]

John Pattison, M.D., and J. Weldon Fell, M.D., of England, successfully treated cancer non-surgically in the mid-1800s, using various chemicals, herbs and poultices.[27] F. W. Forbes Ross, M.D., of London, was one of the first to attempt to systematically correct biochemical imbalances in cancer patients.[28] He placed patients on restricted diets and increased their intake of certain nutrients. Robert Bell, M.D., also advocated dietary therapy for cancer patients in the late 1800s and early 1900s.[29]

In this century, American physicians Lucius Bulkley, M.D., and Charles Ozias, M.D., were well-known proponents of nutritional cancer therapy. Dr. Bulkley, of the New York Skin and Cancer Hospital, was also decades ahead of his time in his diagnosis of cancer through examination of urine, blood and lymphatic secretions.

Naturalistic cancer therapies proposed in the mid- to late-1900s that are still being used by many cancer therapists include those devised by W. B. Coley, M.D., William Koch, M.D., Harry Hoxsey, M.D., Max Gerson, M.D., and Virginia Livingston, M.D.

These therapies are, for the most part, centered around stimulating natural immunity, aiding general systemic function, and improving elimination of toxic and necrotic matter. Some of them, such as the therapy originated by Dr. Livingston, of San Diego, are essentially "immunotherapeutic," meaning that they are primarily concerned with only the immune system. Others, including those used by the metabolic doctors that Dr. W. D. Kelley works with, are concerned with a broader spectrum of all of the body's systems, and are therefore frequently called "metabolic therapies." "Metabolism" refers to one's total energy exchange with the environment. Virtually all of the metabolic therapies contain a nutritional component, as well as one of "detoxification," or internal cleansing.

The history of the vitalistic tradition may be long, but if civilization endures, the vitalistic tradition's future will probably eclipse the tradition's past by many centuries.

CHAPTER SIX

What Really Causes Cancer

What Is Cancer?

The cells of the body are governed by an inborn sense of order. They all possess an innate respect for the rest of the body. When a cell dies, the body strives to replace it with an identical cell. Each of the body's seventy to one hundred trillion cells works for the benefit of every other cell, sometimes sacrificing its own life so that the body as a whole may function and flourish: one for all and all for one.

A cancer cell does not respect these rules. A cancer cell is a selfish renegade, a cell that divides uncontrollably, again and again, until it eventually forms a mass of similar cells that is identified as a malignant tumor.

In a sense, it is surprising that this situation does not occur more often than it seems to, given the immense number of cells in the body. Linus Pauling, in *Cancer and Vitamin C,* puts it this way: "The specialized cells of the gastrointestinal tract, millions and millions of them arranged in fronds and villi to increase their functional area, busily secrete digestive enzymes and absorb the processed nutrients for distribution to their compatriots. They wear out and die and are then discarded, broken down into small molecules for recycling or elimination. They are automatically replaced by fresh, vigorous, young descendants ready to carry on the same function. And yet for most human beings, we do not see an intestine choked and blocked by solid masses of such cells, or a useless intestine completely devoid of them."[1]

The fact that most people never develop discernible tumors is testimony to the body's superb abilities to maintain order and to regain order when it has been temporarily lost.

When this order is lost, though—through growth of a malignant cell—every new generation of the malignant cell is just as "ruthless," just as much the "pirate," as is the initial malignant cell. These generations of cancerous cells travel throughout the body, by way of the bloodstream and lymphatic system, invading masses of normal cells and stealing these cells' nutrients, water, space and oxygen.

Cancer cells have several characteristics that identify them from normal cells. They have larger and more irregular nuclei, which caused cancer cells to be called "monstrous" by the first pathologists to view them after the invention of the microscope. They have an ability to proliferate even when they come into contact with a normal cell; two healthy cells automatically stop reproducing when they touch, as a response to a signal from their membranes. Some cancer cells respirate by means of fermentation, whereas normal cells respirate by oxygenation. Cancer cells, even when they are in the same tumor, can vary in their number of chromosomes, which contain genetic "information." Cancer cells can secrete a substance that causes increased blood flow, and therefore increased nutrition, to the area of the tumor. The primary difference of cancer cells, of course, is that they reproduce uncontrollably. In many ways, then, cancer cells are mutant cells, different in structure and function from healthy cells.

Malignant cell growth is not identified as the disease "cancer" until enough cells have amassed to be an identifiable tumor, or, in leukemias and lymphomas, to disrupt proper function of the circulatory or lymphatic system. Once the disease of cancer is identifiable, it can be measured in stages. The first stage of cancer is a tumor confined to the organ of origin. The second stage is marked by a spread to a nearby lymph gland. Stage three is characterized by a spread to a more distant lymph gland or to an adjacent organ. Stage four is a cancer that has spread to a distant organ, a condition referred to as a "metastasis," which is generally considered incurable.[2]

Death from this disease occurs when the uncontrollably dividing cancer cells impinge upon a vital organ, limiting the function of the organ to a degree that life cannot be sustained. Malignant tumors, per se, do not cause death. A tumor of the liver, though, or lungs, can keep these organs from providing their life-supporting functions. Pain often occurs when malignant cells invade the nerves of tissues and organs, irritating them and stripping away their protective sheaths. Pain also can occur from displacing organs and tissues.

What Causes Cancer?

It is not definitely known why cells begin dividing uncontrollably. The most frequently advanced theory is that the cell loses its genetic "memory." Each cell is "programmed" with a genetic code of information in its nucleus that tells it, among other things, when to divide and when to stop dividing. Cancer cells are often thought to be cells with damaged memories.

A less popular theory of cancer origin, but one that may be valid for some cancers, is the "trophoblastic theory." This theory holds that cancer cells are trophoblasts: simple sex cells, whose normal job is to reproduce rapidly. According to this theory, cancer cells are trophoblasts that are not in their proper site in the body, the sex organs. When these sex cells are not in the gonads, they are thought to lose the biochemical properties that inhibit limitless reproduction, and become, according to this theory, cancer cells.

The "lost memory" theory is the most popular concept of cancer causation, and, it would appear, the one most likely to be true. The entire life-long series of functions of a cell are stored in its "memory," which is found in the cell's genes. Genes are clumped together into groups called chromosomes in a cell's nucleus. In a normal cell there are 46 chromosomes, each of which has 1,800 to 3,000 genes in it. The genes pack away their "memories" in the substance abbreviated as DNA.

Before a cell divides, each gene directs the making of a perfect duplicate of itself. Sometimes, however, not enough "building materials," in the form of nutrients, are available, or an outside force directly impairs the DNA in the chromosomes. Hence, an error is made, and an imperfect cell is manufactured, perhaps one with 45 or 47 chromosomes. This imperfection of succeeding generations of cells is absolutely common, totally predictable. If there were no errors made in generational successions of cells, there would, indeed, be none of the physical deterioration we generally associate with aging. When genetic memory is disrupted, a condition more serious than mere gradual deterioration may occur, however—the cell may lose the information that causes it to stop dividing. When this happens, a cancerous cell can result.

There are other theories that have fewer adherents. One is the viral theory, which attracted enormous attention in the 1960s and 1970s, but is now largely in disrepute. Another is the bacteriological theory, proposed by, among other doctors, Virginia Livingston, M.D., of San Diego.

Dr. Livingston originated the theory that people have a multiform bacterial organism in their blood, tissues, and fluids that can attack the genetic "memory" in the nuclei of healthy cells, causing them to proliferate uncontrollably, rather than reproducing in the normal, controlled manner. However, says Dr. Livingston, white blood cells and antibodies normally keep these bacterial agents to a minimum and kill cells that they have attacked.[3] But when the immune system is weak, the bacteria—which she has named *Progenitor cryptocides*—can take over. The new, maverick cells that are created are coated by a hormone, human chorionic gonadotrophin, which "hides" them from the white blood cells.[4]

Dr. Livingston says these bacterial organisms can be seen through the television screen of a darkfield microscope. They are in abundance in cancer patients, she says, but rare in healthy patients. She says that animals can be given cancer by injecting them with these bacteria.

What Do Carcinogens Do?

Larry Agran, in *The Cancer Connection,* describes the process of cancer causation in the lungs of a steelworker named Joe Fitman: "As it happened, Joe Fitman's principal exposure was in breathing a series of airborne carcinogens that are most reactive with tissue in the respiratory system. These carcinogens were silently, relentlessly bombarding the cells in his bronchial tubes, beginning a process that slowly but irreversibly altered their essential structure. The cells bore a carcinogenic imprint that, in turn, they transmitted to each succeeding generation of cells. Over the years, the normal cells gave way to generations of abnormal cells and, finally, to a generation of cancerous cells: cells targeted and programmed to wreak biologic havoc. Cancerization. Cells, which were once the building blocks of life, give rise to cells that become the opposite of life. Their growth and appetite are uncontrolled. They clump together in tumors. They spread in a crablike fashion, invading adjacent tissue. And then, unchecked, they metastasize; some of these malignant cells break away to be carried in the bloodstream and lymph channels, reaching distant organs where they lodge and grow and spread further. In the end, cancerization means the cell has become the anticell. Life has become antilife. And finally, the body succumbs to the invasion. Death. This is the general outline of the cancerization process."[5]

Most people think that "carcinogen" means "cancer-causing agent." This is not, strictly speaking, correct, as Agran indicates. The things we think of as carcinogens, or cancer-causers, such as cigarette smoke or red dye, are agents that change the structures of chromosomes and interfere with other functions of the cell. They are "mutagenic," meaning that they cause genetic and functional mutation. Substances can be mutagenic without causing cancer, but most substances that can cause a cell to mutate create a process that could result in cancer.

Often, the damage caused by an irritating agent, like the tars in cigarette smoke, can be repaired by the cell. Most people, for example, have an enzyme in their bodies that can repair genetic damage to skin cells. Other mechanisms can repair more generalized damage to these cells. These repairs to the DNA and to the other parts of the cell occur constantly. Sometimes, though, the repairs to the cell are made improperly, and sometimes, because of a weakness in the repair mechanism or a heavy onslaught of damage, complete repairs are not made. When this happens, the weaknesses and errors are repeated in succeeding generations of cells, and can cause anything from slow deterioration of the cell, to death of the cell, to a loss of memory to stop dividing.[6]

Because a cell may take many generations to mutate enough

to become a cancer cell, there is often a long "latency period" between exposure to a gene-damaging substance and onset of malignancy. Thus, many of us probably have "time bomb" cells scattered throughout our bodies.

Industrial powers like tobacco companies and makers of some chemicals often seem to delight in this latency period, since it places a wide time spread between exposure to their product and the onset of cancer, thereby clouding their responsibility in the tragedy. Spokespersons of these companies also frequently remind us that it cannot be said that any particular agent "causes" cancer, but that some merely "promote" it, "contribute to it," or are "associated" or "linked" to cancer. However comforting these euphemisms may be from a legal standpoint, though, it is undeniable that certain substances are at the root of many cancers. Linus Pauling says, "The various 'causes' of cancer represent in fact positive correlations: an increased incidence of cancer is observed to occur in the presence of some substance or circumstance so often as to force us to conclude that there is a cause-and-effect relationship."[7]

Adherents to the genetic damage theory of cancer indict carcinogens as part of cancer causation. The genetic damage theory holds that the carcinogen is the agent of original harm to the chromosomes— that the cigarette smoke, for example, was the substance responsible for scrambling the gene's memory. Carcinogens also promote cancer, according to this theory, by draining the body's repair, recuperative and eliminative potential at the site of irritation.

Whether carcinogens are culprits by destroying cellular memory, or by sapping repair potential, or by doing both, one fact nonetheless remains—wherever there are carcinogens, there is cancer.[8]

Everything Does Not Cause Cancer

A common phrase one hears these days is, "Everything causes cancer." A recent newspaper cartoon showed a white-smocked researcher concluding balefully, "Now we know. *Life* causes cancer." This perception is as destructive as it is false. Everything does not cause cancer. The vast majority of all cancers are caused by only a few basic factors.

Most cancers can be placed in four categories. They are (1) cancers of the lung; (2) cancers of the sex-related organs; (3) cancers of the gastrointestinal tract; and (4) cancers of the "filtering" organs of the body, such as the kidneys, liver and lymph glands. These four categories of cancer account for 90 per cent of all cancer deaths. The causes of these cancers are generally relatively limited. Examined separately, with regard to causation, these four categories of cancer present not a bewildering, complex threat, but four potential problems that can be, with conscientious effort, headed off.

(1) *Lung Cancers.* They are almost always linked with smoke inhalation. Usually the smoke comes from tobacco. Less often it comes from polluted air.[9]

(2) *Cancers of the sex-related organs.* These cancers, including cancers of the uterus, cervix, breasts, testicles and prostate, are usually linked to poor diets, most often diets that are excessively high in animal fat consumption. Poor diets, high in fat, are thought to disturb levels of sexual hormones.[10]

(3) *Cancers of the gastrointestinal tract.* This category includes cancers of the oral-digestive system, including cancers of the lip, mouth, throat, stomach, small intestine, colon and rectum. These cancers are almost always linked to the substances that we habitually put into our systems—what we eat, smoke and drink. The offending substances, according to large-population (or "epidemiological") studies, are excess animal fat, excess processed foods, alcohol, food additives, and tobacco smoke. Of these, excess animal fat appears to be the most harmful, primarily because it is the substance most closely linked to cancers of the colon, which account for the majority of all cancers in this category.[11]

(4) *Cancers of the "filtering" organs.* These cancers, including cancers of the kidney, liver, lymphatic system, gall bladder and pancreas, are usually linked to exposure to toxic chemicals. These cancers are quite often related to one's workplace. Chemical workers, for example, have extremely high rates of these forms of cancer. Cancer of the blood—leukemia—is also related to exposure to toxic chemicals, as well as to exposure to radiation.[12] Because these carcinogens are often airborne and invisible, this category of cancers is the most difficult to prevent.

The remaining forms of cancer include cancers of the eye, brain, bone, and endocrine glands other than the thyroid, and a few other very rare forms of cancer. Of these cancers, brain cancer is the most common, striking less than one per cent of all cancer victims.[13]

There are, of course, cases of cancer that defy the apparent rules of causation—lung cancers, for example, in people who neither smoke nor live in a polluted atmosphere. These exceptions, however, are limited. Smokers have more than ten times as much lung cancer as non-smokers. Similarly, consumers of large amounts of animal fat have ten to twenty times as much chance, compared to consumers of little dietary fat, of contracting cancers of the gastrointestinal tract or sex-related organs, according to epidemiological studies.

It is sometimes said that we live in "a sea of carcinogens." While this is, to some extent, true, we must face up to the fact that most of our exposure to carcinogens is by choice. The most disruptive agents to our health, in terms of cancer, are the cigarettes we choose to smoke and the food we choose to eat. Poor eating habits account for an estimated "60 per cent of all new cancers in women and 40 per cent of all new cancers in men," according to the National Cancer Institute.[14] Tobacco smoking accounts for as much as 25 per cent of all cancer deaths, according to a 1977 report of the U.S. Department of Health, Education and Welfare.[15] The positive aspect of this situation, of course, is that exposure to carcinogens rests, to a great extent, in our own hands.

Carcinogens We Choose To Eat and Smoke

The concept that certain types of diets are associated with cancer was once highly suspect as a theory, but is now considered part of the orthodox view of cancer. This shift in thinking occurred primarily as a response to facts gained from studies of diseases of population sub-groups. These epidemiological studies show that countries with less industrialized food production methods have fewer incidences of cancer. However, when people from these countries immigrate to a country with a highly industrialized food producing industry, these immigrants begin to suffer the same high cancer rates as their new countrymen. This has been proven to occur, for example, in African and Japanese immigrants. It has also been shown that groups in America who eat special diets, lacking in a high degree of processed foods and animal fat, experience much less cancer than the rest of the American population. Among these groups are Seventh Day Adventists.

Laboratory experiments also prove the impact that food has upon cancer incidence. Animal experiments show that certain chemicals, as well as excess amounts of some foods, such as animal fat, cause excess cancer rates in tested animals.

Foods themselves, however, rather than the chemicals added to them, seem to represent the primary cancer threat. Excess fat and processing appears to be more of a danger than chemical additives.

Excess animal fat has been inextricably linked to colo-rectal cancers and cancers of the sex-related organs. Excess fatty acids retard the length of time fecal matter is in the intestines. They also increase the concentration of colonic anaerobic bacteria and, thirdly, increase colonic bile acid secretion. All of these factors are related to incidence of colon cancer, the most common form of cancer in humans.

Excess animal fat consumption also appears to disrupt hormone levels by disturbing endocrine functions. This hormonal upset has been very closely linked to cancers of the breast, uterus, cervix, testes and prostate.

Excessive consumption of processed foods is also linked to colo-rectal cancers. Lack of dietary fiber and high caloric intake, both of which are often present in a highly-processed diet, are strongly related to colon cancers.

Food additives, as well as pesticide and herbicide residue, are also implicated in malignancies. Agents found in foods, such as DES, many brands of herbicides and pesticides, nitrites, dyes and saccharine, are mutagenic and carcinogenic. These agents, some of which have "latency periods" of up to 30 years, disrupt chromosomal balance and create cancerous cells. They also can impede normal metabolic function by overburdening the systems of natural detoxification, such as the liver or lymph glands. Pesticides and herbicides, in particular, have been linked to excessive deaths from cancers of the pancreas, liver and lymph glands, and from leukemia.

Knowing what one should eat is primarily a matter of common sense. A moderate, balanced diet, high in nutrition and low in adulterated, fatty foods, will provide immense protection against cancer.

The significance of smoking in our society is enormous. Smoking constitutes the single most hazardous health habit that any modern civilization has ever chosen to engage in.

More than 3,000 components of tobacco smoke have been identified, and a number have been specifically implicated in cancer. About 90 per cent of cigarette smoke is composed of a dozen gases that are hazardous to health, and the remainder is particulate matter, of which tar and nicotine are the most widely known components.

The particulate matter in tobacco is small enough to reach the furthest recesses of the lungs, and there are about one hundred million of these particles in each cubic centimeter of cigarette. An inhaling smoker retains 70 per cent of the particulates taken in. One of these particulates, condensate of tar, is made up of hundreds of chemicals, some of which are cancer-related.

Besides lung cancer, which kills 80,000 Americans annually, smoking contributes to cancers of the larynx, pharynx, oral cavity, esophagus, pancreas and bladder. Smoking is thought to play a major part in all of these forms of cancer, which kill about 131,000 Americans per year.[16]

In women, who each year have increased their smoking as a group, there has been a 400 per cent increase in lung cancer in the last 30 years. If present trends continue, lung cancer will pass breast cancer within a few years as the major cancer threat to women.

Environmental Carcinogens

Less easily influenced by the individual is exposure to environmental carcinogens, including those that are in the air and water and are present at our job sites. With effort, however, a person can avoid these substances. These chemical carcinogens promote cancers of the "filtering" organs and sometimes the lungs.

The development of synthetic chemicals escalated drastically following World War II. Now the average home is filled with synthetic products, often petroleum-based. Some clinical ecologists (doctors who deal with chemical-caused reactions) say that indoor chemical pollution levels are six to ten times in excess of outdoor pollution levels, due to gas ranges and heaters, pest strips, hair sprays and deodorants, synthetic carpets, drapes and furniture, insulation products, dry cleaning materials, bleaching agents, etc. Many of these products have been shown to disrupt chromosomal arrangements.[17]

Our job sites are as polluted as our homes. Rubber industry workers have shown very high rates of stomach and prostate cancers and leukemia. Steel workers, especially those working above coke ovens, show elevated incidences of kidney and lung cancers. Chemical hazards in the workplace have only very recently begun to receive the attention of unions and governmental protective agencies. Recently exposed hazards that have received special attention are those involving PCB, PCV, asbestos, the pesticide DBCP, uranium and fiberglass. These workplace-related chemicals, the government estimated in 1979, may be responsible for as many as 40 per cent of all cancers, and may take as long as 30 years to result in a clinically diagnosable cancer. Asbestos and fiberglass workers and uranium miners have extraordinarily high rates of lung cancers. Approximately 50 per cent of all uranium miners die of lung cancer. In one study of dye workers, 94 per cent of all workers exposed to dye for five years or longer developed bladder cancer.[18]

Most attempts to limit exposure of workers to toxic chemicals have been quashed by the offending industries, through economic and political maneuvering. The risks of working with asbestos, for example, have been known for decades; not since 1918 have asbestos workers in America or Canada been able to buy life insurance. It was not until 1972, though, that asbestos workers began to receive some protection from the substance they work with.[19]

As the country becomes more urbanized and industrialized, the condition of our air continues to deteriorate. Air pollution has increased approximately 1,200 per cent since 1945. Large, polluted cities have lung cancer rates several times higher than those of areas with clean air, and residents of industrial areas of large cities commonly experience up to ten times the lung cancer rates of less polluted areas of the city.

Over 200 synthetic organic chemicals, many of them known to be harmful to humans, have been identified in drinking water. Toxic substances in water include chloroform, carbon tetrachloride, benzene, vinyl chloride, lindane, aldrin and bischloroethylether. Not until 1974 was a federal clean water law passed, and this was done after it had been shown that the drinking water of New Orleans was exceedingly high in toxic chemicals. The 1974 law limits only ten chemicals in water, however. Several states, including Illinois, have consistently resisted compliance with the law.[29]

The rural setting, once considered the last clean frontier of a polluted society, is now becoming a stockpile site for toxic chemicals, primarily herbicides and pesticides. We are now in the "third generation" of pesticides. The first generation, which lasted until the 1940s, included primarily naturally occurring organic chemicals. The second generation consisted of DDT and related organochlorine pesticides. With this second generation family of herbicides now in disrepute, chemists are struggling to produce chemicals that will not be overly toxic. These "narrow spectrum" insecticides are in their infancy, however, and cancer rates, particularly of bladder and pancreatic cancers and leukemia, are still very high amongst farmers. Many of the pesticides and herbicides become widely dispersed from their primary areas of application, making these substances one of the most lethal general environmental pollutants.[21]

Unfortunately, it is basically up to the individual to protect himself or herself from carcinogenic hazards, because neither industry nor government has shown consistent ability or willingness to effectively counter the problem.

Avoiding these cancer-related environmental agents can be very difficult, though, for an individual. Changing dietary or smoking habits can be hard, but these personal habits are at least subject to an individual's will power. Air, water and industrial pollution generally are not. A person can move or change jobs, of course, but this is normally easier said than done.

The Best Way to Avoid Cancer

Because most people can not remove themselves from modern society's barrage of carcinogens, and because absolutely no one can avoid every single carcinogenic agent, the next step in defeating cancer is one of consummate importance: establishing immune resistance.

Immunity is the most important aspect of resistance to cancer. Maintaining a strong immune system is the best way to prevent cancer. Stimulating natural immunity is the best way to kill tumors.

The concept of using natural immunity to defeat cancer is, as Ralph Moss, formerly of the Sloan-Kettering Institute, writes in *The Cancer Syndrome,* "one of the great hopes of the cancer establishment."[22] The American Cancer Society said in 1980 that immunology held great hope for the future. Many believe, however, that this approach offers far more than hope, and offers it much sooner than the future. They believe that suppressing cancer with the immune response, using a metabolic therapy, is the currently-available most efficient way of addressing the cancer problem.

The idea that the immune system can kill cancer cells is hardly a new one. In the early 1900s, during attempts to transplant tumors from one animal to another, it was discovered that the host animal's immune system would recognize the tumor as a foreign entity and, in rejecting it, destroy the tumor.[23] This discovery produced a wave of enthusiasm. Researchers attempted to develop a vaccination against tumors, but were unsuccessful. In the early days of immunology, the new science was, according to Sir Peter Medawar, a collection of "barefaced empiricisms and embarrassingly silly terminology, a matter of vaccine and anti-sera and skin tests, and not much else."[24]

During World War II, however, a new burst of knowledge spurred the field. In dealing with the voluminous cases of war-caused burn victims, surgeons attempting skin grafts learned much more about the biology of tissue rejection that is caused by immune reaction. During the 1950s, prominent scientists, such as Sir MacFarlane Burner and Dr. Lewis Thomas, showed in immuno-genetic studies that there did indeed exist agents in the human immune system that can kill malignant cells.[25]

The work of immunotherapists and metabolic therapists since that time has proven that patients can be cured with their own recuperative powers.

How the Immune System Works

The immune system is a complex, extremely powerful defense mechanism that constantly protects the body against invasion from foreign microbes, such as viruses, bacteria and parasites, and foreign tissues. People born without functional immune systems must be sealed off in sterile, germ-free compartments of hospitals, forever shielded from the outside world. Most often these people still die, as children, from infection—or from cancer.

The immune system is generally considered to consist of cells called "macrophages," which exist in tissue, and also white blood cells, called "lymphocytes." Both of these types of cells can recognize and kill foreign substances. In a broader sense, any organ that plays a role in protecting or cleaning the body can be considered to have an immune function. Thus, our protective covering of skin, which allows exit of toxic materials, is a factor in our immunity to foreign objects. Likewise, so is the lymphatic system, which cleans the blood, and the liver, which detoxifies harmful chemicals, and the kidneys, which filter poisons out of the body, and acids in the stomach, which can kill bacteria. Even a common action like coughing can be considered an immune reaction, since it serves to remove foreign, toxic materials.

Macrophages and lymphocytes play an especially dramatic role in immunity to cancer. Every day, it is quite likely, these immune agents kill cancer cells in our bodies. This is called the "tip of the iceberg theory." Explained by June Goodfield: "This says that those cancers which are actually manifested represent only a small proportion of those we have or have had, and that the biological purpose of the immune system—its *raison d'etre* —is to recognize and deal with aberrant cells."[26]

Macrophages are known as "scavenger cells." They surround foreign substances and break them down. Macrophages are fixed within tissues but are transported throughout the body in the blood to serve where they are needed. Lymphocytes, which compose 25 to 30 per cent of all white blood cells, originate in the bone marrow. There are two kinds of them, T-cells and B-cells. T-cells travel to the endocrine gland called the thymus, where they mature. They are then stored in the spleen and lymph glands. They can kill foreign cells directly, or by activating other immune mechanisms. B-cells, unlike T-cells, do not act directly upon foreign material. They produce and secrete proteins into the blood that can destroy invaders. The direct attack by T-cells is called "cell-mediated immunity," while the indirect attack of B-cells is called "humoral immunity."

Groups of cancer cells try to block the immune action against them. They react to the attack by slightly changing their structures, often altering the proteins on their surface to make themselves harder to "identify" as foreign agents. Sometimes the T-cells and B-cells combine with cancer cells, ending the immune reaction. Sometimes the immune factors merely "lose the race," arriving at the site too late to match in number and strength the rapidly multiplying cancer cells. The larger a tumor becomes, the more difficult it is for immune agents to identify and destroy the cells that compose it.

"Clearly," writes Dr. John Fahey of U.C.L.A., "the process of immune destruction of tumor cells is not simple. It involves many factors, including availability of blood supply and the ability of the tumor cell to repair and restore its function after damage, as well as the type of immune response that can be locally waged."[27]

The power of the immune system to destroy malignancy is graphically portrayed in people who have had their immune systems depressed by drugs in order to receive organ transplants. The National Institutes of Health, in a study of 8,000 transplant patients, found that these patients suffered from cancer 100 times as much as would be expected. Doctors noted that the cancers in these patients were identical to cancers seen primarily in older people, who invariably have experienced a degeneration of their immune systems as they have aged.[28]

Children with auto-immune diseases—diseases caused by a "self-destructive" immune system—commonly experience excessive rates of cancer when their immune systems are suppressed with drugs.[29]

A final stark portrayal of the importance of natural immunity to cancer is the extremely high incidence of cancer in a strain of mice called the "NZB strain." All of these mice have a defect in their immune systems, which is the only discernible defect in the strain. Every one of these mice, 100 per cent of them, contract cancer.

Cancer and a weak immune system are inseparable. People can live in this "sea of carcinogens" that we have created for ourselves and thrive—cancer-free—if their immune systems are sufficiently powerful.

Enzymes as an Immune Factor

A crucial factor in the body's immunity to cancer is a sufficient supply of pancreatic enzymes. Enzymes, which occur naturally in all living things, are catalysts, or "causers," of chemical reactions. They not only help digest our food, but also to convert nutrients into the chemicals essential for life.

Enzymes perform several critical functions. One is the neutralization of substances that damage chromosomes and promote cancer. Dr. Arthur Upton, former head of the National Cancer Institute, indicated that increased action of "an enzyme system called microcosmal mixed-function oxidase appears to exert a protective effect in detoxifying carcinogens."[30] This function is not only beneficial as a preventive measure, but can be of use therapeutically, by relieving stress on already overburdened organs of detoxification.

Another important function of enzymes is to insure adequate nutrition to the cancer patient. Proper nutrition not only directly affects the immune system, improving its ability to kill cancer cells, but also prevents "cachexia," or gradual wasting away, one of the most common causes of death of cancer patients.

Probably of most importance, though, is the direct antitumoral effect that has been repeatedly observed in patients who have received oral and injectable enzymes. Invariably, cancer patients with significant tumor masses experience a toxic reaction soon after they take enzymes, which is thought by the doctors administering the enzymes to be a result of partial breakdown of tumor mass and subsequent elimination of necrotic tumor material. This reaction is commonly followed by a shrinkage in tumor, often one objectively measurable. Because patients almost always experience this reaction, doctors have learned that the most efficient way to decrease tumor mass is to alternate periods of enzyme application with periods of non-application, during which stress on the organs of elimination can be relieved. In fact, one of the most significant dangers in metabolic anti-cancer programs occurs if a patient uses too many enzymes too quickly, which can cause a severe toxic reaction that can lead to sickness and even to death. More than any other element in a metabolic program, enzymes consistently demonstrate the most potent anti-cancer activity.

Doctors who use enzymes theorize that enzymes exert this dynamic anti-cancer effect by breaking through the tough, protein-coated cancer cell wall. The wall of a malignant cell is relatively less penetrable than that of a healthy cell, and often the immune functions of T-cells, B-cells and macrophages are stymied by this fortress-like structure. Enzymes, though, which digest even the most insoluble proteins during the nutrient-conversion process, seem to be capable of penetrating this strong cell wall. According to many physicians who use enzymes, enzymes, in effect, "digest" this wall, just as they digest many chemical combinations during food digestion.

It is interesting to note that diabetics, who often have enzymatic deficiencies because of the poor function of their pancreases, experience 300 per cent of the normal cancer rate. It is also worth noting that cancer of the pancreas is the most difficult form of the disease to cure with non-metabolic therapies. Of final note is the fact that the small intestine, into which pancreatic enzymes are emptied and become activated, is one of the few places where cancer almost never strikes.

Doctors who work with Dr. Kelley have found that cancer can be predicted with some degree of accuracy by measuring degree of enzyme production and utilization. This indicator seems to be a more accurate indicator of one's proneness to the disease than other more common cancer predictors, such as dietary and smoking habits and family health history.

For more detailed information on the research done on the

relationship between cancer and enzymes, see the chapter entitled "The Power of Food Supplements."

Cancer Causation

Cancer causation, as has been shown, is a combination of two factors: carcinogenic assault on the cells, and weakness of immune factors, including pancreatic enzyme insufficiency. If either side of the equation were totally eliminated, cancer, metabolic physicians believe, would be eradicated. Since both sides, though, can only be influenced by a matter of degree, it is obviously most prudent to attempt to reduce exposure to cancer-promoting agents while striving to improve the function of one's immune system.

If both of these goals are accomplished, one's chances of contracting cancer, say metabolic physicians, will become a minute fraction of the one-chance-in-four that the general population faces.

It is, though, inevitable that many people will continue to contract cancer. For these people, stronger steps will have to be taken to regain total, vibrant health.

These steps, however, can be taken.

CHAPTER SEVEN

Cancer's "Subtle Signals" That Can Save Your Life

Unlike the Ten Commandments, the Seven Warning Signals of Cancer are not written in stone. However mightily conventional wisdom—aided by the American Cancer Society—may labor to uphold the myth that these particular symptoms are the ultimate in early cancer detection, the Seven Signals are of limited practical value. The unfortunate fact of the matter is, the Seven Signals are a classic example of "too little, too late." If the sponsors of these signals were being realistic and honest, they would be compelled to add an eighth "Signal": a massive, festering tumor.

This is not to say that malignancy cannot be determined in its early stages. This can be done, and is being done, by dozens of immune-oriented doctors, including most who work with Dr. Kelley. These doctors monitor cancer existence by biologic assessment, by determining the presence of risk factors, and by discerning certain very early-stage warning signs of cancer that have been identified. These signs generally occur before the appearance of the A.C.S.'s Seven Signals. These determinants, it appears, are largely accurate, and can ascertain malignancy when it is still relatively easy to defeat.

The Failure of the Seven Signals

The essential weakness of the Seven Warning Signals is that they are virtually all indicators of a tumor so large that it is palpable to the touch, visible to the naked eye, or is blocking normal function of one of the vital organs. By the time a tumor is this large, the disease is usually too far advanced to be eradicated by the most common cancer therapies: chemotherapy, surgery and radiation. Because metabolic cancer therapies are generally more powerful malignancy-destroyers than the more common treatments, they can often cause even advanced cancers to regress and disappear. Ironically, therefore, the Seven Signals are of more benefit to patients using metabolic therapies than to those using the "invasive" therapies most often endorsed by the American Cancer Society, which created the Seven Signals. Even so, metabolic therapies achieve significantly better results when applied to a stage of cancer that is truly early, rather than when they are applied to a cancer that has reached the stage of being noticeable by touch or sight.

The veritable deification of the Seven Signals, it seems, has been part of the overall light-at-the-end-of-the-tunnel public stance of the American Cancer Society and National Cancer Institute during the past 20 years. These agencies' official pollyannas of progress have insisted for years that a "checkup and a check" assure one of safety from cancer, when, in fact, neither checking the body for large malignant lumps nor pouring one's hard-earned savings into research significantly improve one's odds. "Clearly, no current therapy of cancer detection," writes former Sloan-Kettering executive Ralph Moss, "is likely to dramatically decrease the death rate from the disease. In fact, there have been many instances in which patients have followed the A.C.S.'s advice, gotten checkups, received approved therapy early in the course of their illness, and still died."[1]

Cancer researcher George Berkley, Ph.D., agrees with Moss. "As far as medical checkups go, while they may do some good in certain cases, more and more evidence is piling up that they are of limited effectiveness at best."[2] Dr. Richard Spark of the Harvard Medical School says that regular checkups provide scant protection against cancer. "As unpleasant as it may sound to those who would like to believe otherwise," he says, "most diseases can be detected only after symptoms appear. . . . Repetitious annual exams of healthy individuals seem to be profitable only for the physician."[3]

Appearance of any of the Seven Signals is predicated upon existence of a sizeable tumor or visible skin cancer. The signals are: a change in bowel or bladder habits (indicating a large tumor in the eliminative organs); a sore that does not heal or an obvious change in a wart or mole (indicating a fully-developed malignant lesion or developed skin cancer); unusual bleeding or discharge from the urinary, genital or digestive tract (indicating hemorrhage caused by ulceration of an invasive tumor); a thickening or lump in the breast or elsewhere (indicating a developed and quite possibly late-stage tumor); difficulty swallowing or indigestion (indicating a tumor obstructing the throat or stomach or blocking nerve function to the throat); or a nagging cough or hoarseness (indicating malignant growth in the lungs or a tumor causing compression of the nerve to the larynx).[4]

Obviously, these signals do not indicate malignancies in the earliest stages, when they are microscopic collections of cancer cells, or even, in a great many cases, when they are still small and confined to a single site. By the time tumors are apparent to the touch or the eyes, many have spread, or "metastasized." *New York Times* science writer Jane Brody points out that "half of all cancers, excluding cancers of the blood-forming organs, develop metastases during their 'hidden' life before they produce symptoms that would prompt the average person to visit a doctor."[5] Cancer researchers Bangle and Levin concur in an article in the journal *Cancer:* ". . . it is clear that fully invasive cancers can sometimes emerge after little or no preliminary warning."[6]

One of the most common Seven-Signal-based methods of cancer detection is manual manipulation of the breasts, or breast palpation. Long revered as one of the pillars of the Seven Signal detection methods, breast palpation is an excellent example of the inadequacy of the Seven Signals. Even Dr. Philip Strax's pro-palpation book, *Early Detection,* admitted that, "Indeed, there had been mass screening examinations at cancer-detection centers, using clinical examination (palpation) only, with very little effect on the mortality rate. Something else was needed."[7] Dr. Strax discusses a study that tested the effectiveness of breast palpation combined with x-ray. "Much to the surprise of everyone, one-third of the cancers found in the Health Insurance Plan study were not felt by the clinician. At the same time, two-fifths of the cancers were noted by the surgeon, but not detected by the radiologist. In only one-fifth of the cases were the cancers found by both physicians."[8] Strax indicates that to be palpable, the cancer, which may already have metastasized, must either be large, or be close to the surface, or be in a small breast, or be in a breast with little fatty tissue (which is not common in older women, who have the highest rates of the disease). He also states that approximately one-third of all breast cancers begin in the milk ducts and do not produce palpable lumps.[9]

The same problems apply to feeling-detection of other cancers. Cancers in the bowel can be recognized digitally, but there are a multitude of ways to fail to notice the tumors. Tumors in the ovary may actually be as large as softballs and remain unnoticeable to the touch.[10]

Besides not being clearly noticeable to the touch or sight in the very early, mid-growth or even late stages, cancer often gives off ambiguous signals. Researcher John Cairns writes that only one-fifth of a percent of men develop prostate cancer, while 15 per cent to 20 per cent show the symptoms associated with the disease. Likewise, the majority of men in equatorial climates show skin lesions that seem to be precancerous, but only a small minority of these lesions actually become cancer.

Marvelous Mechanistic Misapplications

Presumably bolstering these rather arbitrary and ineffective Seven Signals are an array of mechanistic medical procedures that are generally considered to be capable of making a more totally positive identification of cancer in its earliest stages. Sometimes these procedures are applied after a tumor is felt or seen by the patient; sometimes they're applied prior to personal detection. Among the mechanical means are: biopsy, mammography, thermography, x-ray, proctosigmoidoscopy, ultrasound, laboratory analysis of sputum from the lungs, and papanicolaou tests (or PAP smears).

Unfortunately, these tests, like the Seven Signals, also provide only scant vigilance against cancer. Sometimes they even cause cancer.

Mammography, one of the commonest of the tests, demonstrates the weaknesses of the mechanical methods. The most extensive use of mammography, or x-ray examination of the breast, occurred in the mid-1970s, when the National Cancer Institute and American Cancer Society sponsored a massive free screening program for breast cancer, using primarily mammography. Though the American Cancer Society director boasted at the time that the project was "the greatest PR thing the N.C.I. and A.C.S. have ever done,"[11] the program was an unmitigated flop. Science writer Ruth Rosenbaum investigated the project and concluded that it "showed absolutely no benefit to women under 50, who made up 85 per cent of the program participants."[12] She pointed out that the x-rays promoted future cancers in many of the 270,000 women who participated, and that a significant number of women had their breasts amputated needlessly because of errors in interpreting the test results.[13] Thermography, a study of heat patterns in the breast, is a safer procedure, but almost one woman in every five shows abnormalities in heat concentrations in the breast, making the test inconclusive.

PAP smears are another "sacred cow" that receive more credit than they deserve. Because deaths from uterine and cervical cancers began to decline at almost the same time PAP smears were created, the test has been associated with decreased mortality from the diseases. Even a cursory glance at the epidemiological studies, however, shows that these diseases began to decline somewhat before the test was instituted. *Science* magazine referred to PAP smears as "an idea whose time has gone."[14] In 1979 the American Cancer Society, longtime champions of the procedure, dropped their recommendation for the annual PAP smear, recommending instead one every three years for women aged 20 to 65. The A.C.S. now says that a PAP smear is helpful every three years for women under 20 only when they are sexually active. The tests are not conclusive, are influenced by factors other than cancer, and can be misinterpreted, sometimes causing needless drastic action.

Biopsy, one of the commonest procedures for determining cancer, is useless for screening of large population groups, determines only tumorous, rather than malignant, conditions, does not determine the site of any possible metastasis, can only be used after a tumor has already been located, and fails to determine the size and weight of the tumor. Dictating even more strongly against reliance upon biopsy, though, is the fact that biopsy can spread a tumor and also depress immunity. "Needle biopsy," reports the textbook *Clinical Oncology for Medical Students and Physicians,* may result in ". . . a needle track that may harbor nests of cells which may form the basis for a later recurrent spread. Incisional biopsy of certain highly malignant tumors through an open operative field may be contraindicated because of risk of spread of tumor through the operative field."[15] This textbook also says that biopsies can cause "surgical trauma that decreases natural host resistance of the formation of metastases."[16]

Currently popular medical tests for lung cancer and colon cancer, the most common of all cancers, are also less than effective. Dr. Charles Moertel, director of oncology at the Mayo Clinic, surveyed a study of the most common detection method of colon and rectal cancer—visual examination with a proctoscope—and concluded that "the truly routine proctoscopic evaluation does not seem to be a practical screening test."[17] The American Cancer Society in 1980 abandoned its recommendation that people over 40 have an annual proctosigmoidoscope exam, and also said that there was no reason for people to annually have their stools examined.[18]

The tests for lung cancer—x-rays and examination of sputum (mucus and saliva)—were also denigrated by the A.C.S. in 1980. The society dropped a recommendation that high-risk groups have annual chest x-rays and sputum examinations, saying that "there is actually evidence from a half-dozen studies that such early detection does not reduce mortality."[19] "Very early lung cancers are generally not visible on a chest x-ray," writes the *New York Times'* Jane Brody. "By the time the vast majority of lung cancers produce clear-cut symptoms—chest pain or blood-tinged sputum—the cancer is already well-advanced, with only a seven per cent chance of cure."[20]

Pancreatic cancer is also very hard to detect with conventional means. It is, says Dr. Linus Pauling, "notoriously difficult to diagnose because the symptoms are so vague."[21] Cancer of the pancreas, says Jane Brody, does not "produce readily detectable signs or symptoms until the disease is well advanced. . . ."[22]

The Rise and Fall of Early Detection

The whole thrust of the early detection program, oriented around the Seven Signals and mechanical detection devices, has been seriously blunted of late, simply because it is an ineffective program. The American Cancer Society took a position in 1980 that periodic checkups for all cancers in general were unnecessary.[23]

A valid question is: why did this notion of the importance of early detection through these means enjoy such currency for so long? Ralph Moss, former assistant director of public affairs at America's most famous cancer hospital, Sloan-Kettering, suspects that economics played a part. He wrote recently in *The Cancer Syndrome,* "Cancer diagnosis is a huge medical business, fanned by the public's fear of the disease and 30 years of publicity by the American Cancer Society." Moss believes one of the cornerstones of the early detection program, the PAP smear, was a money-oriented gimmick. "According to two scientists from New York University and the Yale University School of Medicine," wrote Moss, "the annual PAP smear has become so entrenched in this country partly because it has been so heavily promoted and partly because so much of the cost is borne by the private individual. In England and Canada, where the governments bear practically all the costs, annual tests are not recommended. . . ."[24]

Probably as strong a motivator as finances, though, was merely the fact that with cure rates for cancer as poor as they have been, early detection must have seemed a reasonable straw to grasp at in the search for a way out of the cancer miasma.

Just because the previously popular methods of early detection have essentially failed, though, doesn't mean that early detection is a dead-end street.

There are methods of early detection that are effective.

The Real Warning Signals of Cancer

Cancer can be anticipated and recognized in its earliest stages, but this can be done only when the disease is recognized as a failure of systemic function, rather than as a tumor that one can see or touch. If cancer is perceived of as only being existing large lumps, there can be no hope of early detection; this concept of cancer, which is medicine's most common perception of the disease, limits early detection by its very definition.

Cancer must be seen as a slowly-forming condition caused by a combination of health insults and immune weakness in order to "get the jump" on the disease. The best approach to recognizing cancer while it is still in its microscopic stage is (1) to regularly assess the insults one subjects one's health to; (2) to monitor the body's biologic functions; and (3) to be aware of cancer's more subtle warning signals. This overall approach is carried out by use of several health-monitoring exams, including various metabolic physicians' patient evaluation procedures, the "Enzyme Test," the "Navarro," "Schandl" and "Beard" tests, and by simply being aware of one's health and habits.

Metabolic Physicians' Evaluation Procedures

Indexing the insults to one's health, and the body's apparent reactions to these insults, is a highly valuable tool in becoming aware of early cancers. This method, performed as part of patient evaluation procedures, including those conducted by physicians who work with Dr. Kelley, does not identify cancer, but rather assesses the possibility of the disease's presence. Other similar health-assessing tests are given by other doctors and clinics.

For many years, cancer's causes were thought analagous to Winston Churchill's description of Russia: "a riddle wrapped in a mystery inside an enigma." While there is still doubt about the exact mechanisms of malignant formation, we now know that almost all cancers occur because of various health insults. The head of the National Cancer Institute said in 1979 that upwards of 90 per cent of all cancers were directly related to definable, specific health insults, primarily poor diet, tobacco use and exposure to toxic agents.[25]

Identification of these factors has become so precise that a known impact of an offending agent can be realistically considered an indicator, or even precursor, to possible cancer. For example, uranium miners, it is now known, face a 50 per cent chance of contracting lung cancer. If they are also heavy smokers, they face a 90 per cent chance of contracting lung cancer.[26] Similarly it is known that workers in contact with benzidine and betanaphthylamine for approximately five years have a 94 per cent probability of developing cancerous bladder tumors.[27] Using information like this, it can be predicted with considerable accuracy whether a person is likely to be close to having a malignant condition.

These predictions are made by computer analysis of the responses to numerous questions and the results of clinical testing, which compose various doctors' patient evaluation procedures. These procedures ascertain the various risk factors a person has been subjected to, the degree of exposure, the length of exposure, the multiplied threat posed by combinations of risk factors, and signs from the body that the health insult has reduced function of an organ or gland, or has mutated cells. These procedures also measure the ability of the body to recoup from the health insults. By asking so many questions about so many areas of health, immunity and metabolism, and by relying upon proven information about factors that lead to cancer and to immune stress, the weak organs, systems and glands in the body can be targeted. With astounding accuracy, the likelihood of presence of a developing malignancy can be determined. Although a malignancy may not currently exist, it may become apparent from studying results of these procedures that if certain practices or habits are continued, one is likely to develop.

This method of testing is, in a sense, futuristic, insofar as it is a relatively recent endeavor in medicine and does appear to represent the wave of the future. On the other hand, it is little more than the careful application of common sense. Is it really so "magical," when you stop to think about it, that one could predict lung cancer in a heavy-smoking uranium miner who has a chronic cough and shows little immune resistance to common ills?

Exceptions exist to the common risk factors, of course. Ten per cent of heavy-smoking uranium miners do not contract lung cancer. But these people generally show strong immune strength, often are bolstered by factors such as superior nutrition or a genetic background showing good health, or exhibit other positive tendencies which can be spotted in the patient evaluation procedure.

Doctors have, of course, predicted problems through this procedure that have been averted. This is the function of the procedure—to recognize danger and to take the appropriate steps to nullify it.

Thousands of people, by 1981, have used patient evaluation procedures, providing doctors with a wealth of information on risk factors associated with cancer, and upon early indicators of the disease. While the results of a patient evaluation procedure are not intended to be and do not constitute a diagnosis, these results are extraordinarily helpful in making assumptions about malignancies which may not yet be clearly detectable by touch or sight.

I Knew It!

Sometimes when people learn that they may have a malignant condition, doctors report that they can practically see a "light bulb go on in the patients' heads." The patients say, "Oh! Maybe that's why I've felt the way I have lately!"

Cancer generally doesn't strike as a tumor without quietly announcing itself first as a general metabolic condition. Doctors who work with Dr. Kelley have compiled their own warning signals for cancer, which they believe indicate presence of cancer before it has reached the stage of being a palpable or visible tumor, and, therefore, before it can be detected by the A.C.S.'s Seven Warning Signals.

Dr. Kelley, in seminars he gives for physicians, often describes his own symptoms that preceded malignancy. Following is an excerpt from one of his presentations.

"When I had cancer I went through profound changes, none of which were linked by my internist to cancer, but which, in hindsight, clearly were associated with the disease. Since we have begun working with cancer patients, we've found that there are a number of signs that can betray the first stages of cancer. Some of these signs are caused by existence of a tumor, and some are caused by the metabolic changes that people developing cancer commonly experience. Almost no cancer patient we've talked to has not experienced one or more of these indicators, or ones similar to them. It is our opinion that very few people go directly from a state of feeling totally healthy to a state of overt malignancy.

"I now am certain that I had cancer for more than three years before I was diagnosed as having it. One of the first signs I showed of the condition that I believe led to my pancreatic tumor was chronic indigestion and flatulence. A few months later I began to have visual problems, even though I was only 35. I was prescribed bifocals. My third symptom was muscular aches and pains, against which I finally had to apply muscle relaxants. The painful feelings shifted to my chest, so a series of electrocardiograms were taken. A severe state of depression gradually encroached upon me. For months I was tired, unambitious and depressed. I soon started having a hard time concentrating, and was sometimes irrational. My hair began to become dry and brittle.

"Finally, after enduring these symptoms for several years, I was diagnosed as having cancer. By the time the cancer was clinically discovered, it was supposedly too late.

"I now see that the symptoms I'd experienced were classic alarm signals of a developing malignancy, most of which were associated with metabolic disorder rather than tumor growth. The indigestion, for example, was caused by weakness of my liver, pancreas and stomach, which severely lessened my ability to receive the nutrients my immune system so desperately needed, and which decreased my body's ability to detoxify my system. The irrationality, loss of concentration and hair damage were manifestations of my inability to metabolize protein. My brain and hair were not receiving adequate amino acids and other nutrients with which to function correctly, probably because I wasn't secreting enough protein-digesting enzymes, or because my enzymes were being diverted to malignant cells, in my body's attempt to break through the tough malignant cell wall. We have since found that premature graying of the hair, as well as hernias, can also be signs of lack of protein in the hair or muscles. My depression was almost certainly caused by toxicity in my body; malignancies exude toxins that create cerebral dysfunction, including depression. My eyesight suffered, I believe, as a response to lack of nutrients, including protein, and to the generally stressful effects of the developing disease. The cramps in my muscles and chest were the result of depleted calcium in my bloodstream, another manifestation of inability to convert nutrients.

"In my case, after a point, the malignancy in the pancreas was causing these nutritional and enzymatic problems. In most cancer patients, though, nutritional and enzymatic problems, often caused by pancreatic malfunction, allow the malignancy to develop. A poorly functioning pancreas is always an excellent indicator of malignant threat, because of the extreme importance of pancreatic enzymes in breaking down cancer cell walls.

"We are not advising, of course, that everyone with brittle hair or indigestion assume the worst and check into a cancer ward. That would be against the spirit of the proper use of these indicators. If one has indigestion, one should try to improve it with diet, supplements, stress reduction, etc. The proper spirit of using these indicators of health is to employ them as tools to improve general well-being, rather than to fixate upon them as forecasters of malignant doom.

"A good, if rather simplistic, rule of thumb for early diagnosis of cancer is: if you feel great and know you are living a healthy lifestyle, you probably don't have cancer, and probably won't have it soon. The person who is chronically ill with colds and flu, frequently depressed for no apparent reason, and has problems with digestion, assimilation and toxicity, is the person who should be concerned. This person is degenerating systemically, and will, in all likelihood, suffer from a degenerative disease, whether it's cancer, heart disease, arthritis or diabetes. There are exceptions to this rule, of course, but the rule usually holds true."

Biologic Tests for Cancer

A person who is suffering from a combination of the subtle signals that metabolic doctors feel precede a fully-developed malignancy, or whose patient evaluation procedures indicates a proneness to cancer, or who has noticed presence of one of the A.C.S.'s Seven Signals, may choose to biologically monitor his or her body for possible cancer.

This can be done with invasive, mechanistic measures, such as x-ray or biopsy, which may be prudent in many cases. The risks associated with these measures may be outweighed by a need for the information they may provide.

More compatible with the holistic philosophy, though, are two malignancy tests that are sometimes disparaged by mechanistically-oriented physicians. These are the Beard Anthrone Test and the Navarro Immunological Test. There is no proof that these tests are accurate, and, indeed, occasionally, they may be misleading. However, many metabolic doctors' experiences with them has led these doctors to trust them as much as the highly mechanical measures.

Like certain universally accepted tests for prostate cancer, these two tests are blood and urine tests. The Beard test, created in the 1950s by Howard Beard, Ph.D., formerly of Western Reserve University, is an assessment of a person's levels of human chorionic gonadotrophin (HCG), a hormone that is broken down by the pancreatic enzyme chymotrypsin. The Navarro test is another version of the Beard test, created by cancer specialist Manuel D. Navarro, M.D. The tests were shown to be helpful in the detection of malignancy by a radio-immunoassay study conducted by Braunstein in 1973, and by experiments by J. E. Dailey and P. M. Marcuse in 1969.[28]

A related and more sophisticated test, called the "CA Profile," has been recently developed by Dr. Emil Schandl, a biochemist who heads the CA Laboratory, Center for Metabolic Disorders, in Dania, Florida. Dr. Schandl published a report on his test in the July 1980 issue of the *Journal of the American Association for Clinical Chemistry.* The Profile consists of four indicators; Dr. Schandl has written that at least one of the four indicators was found elevated in 94 per cent of patients with documented clinical cancer. The four indicators are all from blood specimens.

The first is the "beta" chain of the human chorionic gonadotrophin hormone, which is also the basis of the Beard and Navarro tests (as well as the familiar pregnancy test). Testing of Beta HCG in blood is done at many hospitals and by many doctors in order to monitor certain sex-related cancers, such as embryonal cell carcinoma and choriocarcinoma.

The second indicator measured in the CA profile is an enzyme, abbreviated PHI, which stands for phospho-hexose-isomerase. This enzyme is important in non-oxygen respiration, which is how many cancer cells continue to live. Schandl has found that elevated levels of PHI in the blood generally indicate a spreading cancer.

The third component of the Profile is the monitoring of another enzyme, abbreviated GGTP, which stands for gamma-glutamyl-transpeptidase. This enzyme is related to liver function. Any overload on the liver will cause an increased release of this enzyme.

The fourth measurement of the profile is abbreviated CEA, which stands for carcino-embryonic antigen. The discovery of this substance over a decade ago was accompanied by much excitement, because many researchers thought that finally a single reliable blood test for cancer had been found. The test contains some ambiguities, however, although it has proved to be a useful indicator of response to therapy in cancers of the digestive tract, liver and pancreas.

All of these biological tests are often capable of detecting malignant cell growth in its earliest stages. They can be of benefit as mass-screening techniques, they differentiate between benign and malignant tumors, they are absolutely safe, and they are inexpensive. The shortcomings of these tests are that they sometimes fail to recognize some liver cancers, can be affected by pregnancy, can be ambiguous because of other factors, and fail to determine the type or location of the malignancy.

Details on these tests can be received from, among other informational agencies, the Cancer Control Society of Los Angeles, or the Foundation for Alternative Cancer Therapies of New York City.

Metabolic doctors do not claim that these tests are the ultimate diagnostic procedures, but, rather, that they are helpful educational tools.

The Enzyme Test

One of the simpler and more revealing tests developed in the past 15 years is the Enzyme Test, which is simply administration of a rather heavy dose of pancreatic enzymes to a person suspected of having an existing tumor. The most effective time to administer the test appears to be when the cancer is six to 36 months old, a time span during which cancer is often undetectable through mechanistic tests or by touch or sight.

Doctors advise taking eight high-quality enzyme tablets after each meal for four weeks. A low-quality product can render the test ineffective.

If a person feels noticeably worse within four weeks after

beginning the enzymes, there is a possibility that a mass of malignant cells has been killed and has produced a toxic reaction. The negative feelings of the toxic reaction may include nausea, swelling of the lymph glands, a feeling of general malaise, and lack of energy.

If a person feels more energetic and in a stronger emotional and mental condition than he or she has recently felt, following the ingestion of the enzymes, it may be that he or she has a precancerous condition, one associated with pancreatic deficiency, which the enzymes help to compensate for.

If there is no noticeable reaction to the enzymes, there is, in all probability, no existing tumor mass or pancreatic deficiency.

The test should be repeated every six months.

The enzyme test is safe, provides very early indication, can be an effective mass screening tool, differentiates between benign and malignant tumors, and does not spread the disease. The disadvantages of the test are that it does not determine type, size or site of the tumor, it is more expensive than the urine tests, it can fail to indicate a very large, difficult-to-penetrate tumor, and can be ineffective if the liver is functioning very poorly.

Again, this test is not considered the sole worthy evaluative technique that one might wish to employ, but is thought to be another valuable learning experience.

Early Detection

If the heretofore most common methods of early detection have been proven lackluster of late, the newer methods appear to be on the ascent.

Early detection is a very promising field, but it only reaches its peak of dependability when it is performed with an adequate knowledge of risk factors, of physical and mental clues to early malignancy, and of responses of the body to certain biologic tests.

Searching the body for large tumor masses has, it would appear, never really been a method of "early" detection, even though this method was promoted as one. The body can apparently be "searched" in inordinately more sophisticated ways.

This early discovery of cancer can lead to early treatment, which is invariably the most profitable to the patient—*if it is the right kind of treatment.*

CHAPTER EIGHT

The Common Therapies: Positive and Negative Aspects

In 1976 Benjamin Byrd, M.D., then president of the American Cancer Society, wrote in *American Legion* magazine that "the rate of long-term survival for early cancers is 85 to 99 per cent, as against only 53 per cent in the case of advanced tumors."[1] The fact that this man, occupying the position he did at that time, could get away with a statement so fundamentally untrue, is testimony to the veracity of an undeniable truth: nothing is easier than telling people what they want to hear.

The people Dr. Byrd made this statement to may well have found comfort in the doctor's inflated survival figures, for the truth in this matter is a harsher verdict to accept: at most, 33 per cent to 40 per cent of all early cancers are commonly cured, and no more than one per cent of all late-stage cancers are commonly cured, according to the 15th edition of the *Encyclopedia Britannica* and most medical sources, including the National Cancer Institute.[2]

Dr. Byrd, however, is hardly the only culpable figure in the misleading of the American public on response rates to chemotherapy, surgery and radiation as treatments for malignancy. Virtually every A.C.S. publication tries to paint a patina of progress on cancer therapy by stressing the few notable advances occurring in recent cancer therapy. The A.C.S.'s 1980 "Cancer Facts and Figures," for example, tells us that "some tumors, formerly with very poor prognoses, now are being cured in many cases." The booklet assures us that "surgery is now more precise," that "50 drugs have been found effective against cancer and others being tested appear to hold promise," and that "certain drugs and hyperthermia are being used to increase the effectiveness of radiotherapy."[3] The A.C.S. happily refers to cancer as "the most curable of diseases." One might well infer that the "light at the end of the tunnel" is in full, incandescent view, and that good-old American know-how has tumors on the run. Would it were so.

Unfortunately, there has been little improvement in cancer cure statistics since the mid-1930s, with the notable exception of those gained with metabolic, immunotherapeutic approaches, which fewer than five per cent of all cancer patients are well-informed enough to seek out. There was a slight 13 per cent improvement in the overall cancer cure rate from the mid-1930s until the mid-1950s, but, according to researcher Seymour Epstein, M.D., "The modest improvement from the 20 per cent overall five-year survival rates in the mid-1930s to 33 per cent in the mid-1950s reflects advances in surgery, blood transfusion, and antibiotic treatment, rather than specific advances of cancer treatment."[4]

The 1930's rate is even a highly dubious figure, since it is an extrapolation of the rates from just one state, Connecticut. No national statistics were compiled at that time. A recent director of the Connecticut Tumor Registry said that Connecticut's figures may not accurately mirror the nation's, because the state is demographically different from the rest of the country.

Since 1960, not even the general advances in medicine have been enough to bolster cancer's survival rates. "Over the last two decades," writes Dr. Epstein in *The Politics of Cancer,* "there has been no further significant improvement in overall cancer survival rates."[5] There is general agreement in the medical community that cancer survival rates have increased only approximately two per cent since 1940.[6] Since there have been significant life-extenuating general advances in surgical procedures and in crisis care intervention, it may be true that most common therapies are actually less effective now than they were 30 or 40 years ago.

"Modern figures on cancer survival rates are not encouraging," writes Dr. Epstein. "When the percentage of people who have survived five years after cancer diagnosis and treatment in the period 1965-1969 are compared to similar figures for 1950-1969, it can be seen that with the exception of Hodgkin's disease, cancer of the prostate and some relatively uncommon cancers such as acute lymphocytic leukemia, choriocarcinoma, and Wilm's tumor, no substantial overall progress has been made in treating cancer."[7]

The successes in the rare, obscure forms of the disease are much-trumpeted. Rare is the A.C.S. pamphlet that does not refer to advances in Wilm's tumor or acute lymphocytic leukemia. But this meager success is dwarfed by the fact that the most common cancers, those that have always accounted for almost nine of every ten cancer deaths, are almost as impervious to the common treatments as ever. The survival rates for lung and colon cancers have improved one per cent in the past 30 years, survival with breast cancer has increased four per cent, and survival with cervical cancer has decreased by three per cent. Lung cancer, according to the American Cancer Society's "Cancer Facts and Figures," still kills, within five years, 90 per cent of all those who contract it, just as pancreatic cancer kills about 95 per cent, liver cancer kills about 90 per cent, esophageal cancer kills about 90 per cent, bone cancer kills about 95 per cent, breast cancer kills about 50 per cent, stomach cancer kills about 88 per cent, colon cancer kills about 50 per cent, and leukemia kills about 50 per cent.

The Textbook of Medical Surgical Nursing recently estimated that 85 per cent of all people with all forms of cancer, both early and late-stage, will die of the disease. This same figure has been used by former National Cancer Institute Director Dr. Frank Rauscher and the Mayo Clinic's Dr. Charles Moertel. About half of these patients die within one year of their initial diagnosis.[8]

An 85 per cent death rate does not seem to indicate progress. If this is progress, then what constitutes a stalemate?

Cancer's Public Relations

In 1975 the American Cancer Society issued a report claiming that "cancer incidence has declined slightly in the last 25 years." This, of course, was welcome news to the American public, since it contradicted what most people had been thinking—that cancer incidence had risen alarmingly. Investigator Ruth Rosenbaum, however, uncovered the real reason for this proclaimed "decline." In an interview with A.C.S. vice president Irving Rimer, Rimer admitted to Rosenbaum that "somewhere around 1972 or 1973, we stopped including in our calculations all skin cancers except melanoma, the only one that's fatal, and also *in situ* cervical cancers, because many experts don't consider these to be cancers at all."[9]

Rimer conceded that since minor skin cancers and cervical cancers occur in the hundreds of thousands every year, the sudden exclusion of these diseases from the statistics had in fact accounted for this alleged "decline" in cancer.

Sadly, this example of reconstructing facts and figures to fill propaganda needs has been more the rule than the exception with the A.C.S. and National Cancer Institute. "It is this type of outright dishonesty and statistical legerdemain that supports the country's system of orthodox cancer treatment and leads the public to believe that the medical establishment is well on the way to controlling cancer," writes Rosenbaum.[10]

Another example of A.C.S. story-telling is their 1975 claim that 1,500,000 Americans were then alive who had had cancer, a figure that included those with skin and cervical cancers. They were forced to drop this grand total by their chief statistician, who considered it founded on an unreliable data base, but then boldly upped the number to two million the next year, possibly by including some of the half-million new cancer patients of that year, many of whom hadn't died yet.

The cancer cure rates promoted by the A.C.S. and N.C.I. are suspect for various reasons. One is that they don't really represent cures, but merely people who are alive five years after diagnosis. It is utterly common for a person to die more than five years after treatment, a dead celebrant of a cancer "cure." In general, about half of all cancer patients die between their fifth and tenth year after diagnosis. In cancers of the kidney, lung and stomach, more than half die of cancer after the fifth year following diagnosis.[11] By this token, cancer "cure" rates, low as they are, are really only about half as high as they appear.

Another factor that makes the rates look better than they are is the fact that only about a dozen cancer hospitals, all of them major research centers in large cities, contribute to the official cancer statistics. The approximately three per cent of all cancer patients treated at these hospitals receive the best technological care that is available. It has been shown that some of the poorer hospitals have cancer death rates twice as high as those of the best hospitals.[12] A great many of the patients treated at the poor hospitals are non-white; the non-white cancer death rate is approximately 300 per cent higher than the death rate for white people.

Another device used to sugar-coat cancer statistics is the use of the word "respond," implying a movement toward cure. The A.C.S. and N.C.I., for example, claim that "about one-third of all cancers are responding to chemotherapy." To this claim, Dr. Marvin Zelen of the Eastern Cooperative Oncology Group, which specializes in clinical trials of drugs, replied: "It depends on what you mean 'responding.' You have to distinguish between cure and a very temporary response."[13]

Why would the A.C.S. and N.C.I. attempt to gloss over this devastating problem? Most probably, they do so to perpetuate the strength of their own organizations and that of the mutually-supportive technological medical community. "The basis of A.C.S. propaganda," says medical/political analyst Peter Barry Chowka, "is provided by statistics which are cited in an attempt to show impressive improvements in cancer survival rates due to intervention of expensive, symptomatic chemical and technological treatments."[14]

The National Cancer Institute, like any other governmental agency, may feel, with some justification, that its funding potential exists in direct proportion to its ability to solve its assigned task—or, failing that, to appear to solve it.

The American Cancer Society, which depends on donations, has found that people will not give money to a hopeless cause. Barbara Culliton, of *Science* magazine, attended an annual A.C.S. pre-fund-drive press extravaganza, which every year generates hundreds of optimistic stories about cancer therapy. "A.C.S. assumes," she surmised, "that if people are exposed to good news about cancer shortly before a society volunteer comes knocking at your door, donations will be highest."[15]

This may be a good marketing technique, but, it is really not fair to the American medical consumer.

Surgery, Radiology and Chemotherapy

"Cut, burn and poison" therapy is an unkind euphemism for surgery, radiation and chemotherapy. But the therapies themselves are often unkind. These therapies have shortened life, caused disfigurement, and produced pain, sickness and future illness.

It would be less than reasonable to claim that these therapies are never useful for cancer. Surgery can be very effective in removing minor skin cancers, and achieves 70 per cent five-year survival in uterine cancers. Radiation is frequently effective for lymphosarcoma, can cure over half the men with inoperable, local prostate cancer, and can achieve five-year remission in 80 per cent of very early Hodgkin's disease patients. It can also, as was shown in the first four chapters of this book, help patients survive while their immune systems are being stimulated. Chemotherapy can cure about two-thirds of the women suffering from the rare tumor choriocarcinoma, and can achieve five-year survival rates in about two-thirds of the cases of the relatively rare cancer lymphoblastic leukemia, which is the "showcase" disease for chemotherapy.

Other than these relatively limited successes in mostly rare cancers, though, chemotherapy, surgery and radiation have, for the most part, been failures.

These approaches are failures for two primary reasons: (1) they are largely unsuccessful, and (2) they cause suffering.

Problems with the Common Therapies

Surgery is the therapy that most often helps achieve five-year remissions, mostly because it is the therapy most often applied to localized cancers. The success statistics of surgery, however, don't include those operations in which surgery is performed but no tumor is removed, because of its site or size. The statistics also do not include patients who die within 30 days of the operation; these deaths, credited to postoperative reaction, are common.[16]

Successes credited to surgery are often actually due to a combination of surgery and natural immunity. Although surgeons routinely tell cancer patients that they've "gotten it all," studies have shown that in 25 to 60 per cent of patients, some cancer cells have been left behind after the operation.[17] It is the task of the immune system to kill these cells. Dr. Lucien Israel, consultant to the N.C.I., writes in *Conquering Cancer* that "surgery alone does not radically alter the natural history of cancers."[18] Dr. Israel explains that surgery only "brings the disease back to an earlier point in time," allowing natural immune response to attack the tumor cells.[19] Dr. Israel indicates that 80 per cent of all cancer deaths after surgery result from a growth at a distant site, and admits that "even if we were able to perfect local treatment . . . that would still leave 80 per cent of failures."[20]

Even surgical procedures designed to eradicate cancers that have spread, such as the "Whipple" technique for pancreatic cancer, or "Halstead's radical" mastectomy for breast cancer, are generally ineffective. The Whipple technique, which removes organs adjacent to the pancreas, has a zero to three per cent survival rate for metastasized cancers. Radical breast surgery involving extensive organ, muscle and lymph removal was proven by Dr. George Crile to be no more effective than a less destructive form of the operation, and is now losing popularity.[21]

If surgery, with all its shortcomings, is the most successful cancer therapy, radiation has less to offer. Radiation, used on about half of America's cancer patients, is still considered by many medical people to be a highly dubious endeavor. "Apart from Hodgkins disease and lymphosarcoma," writes Dr. Israel, "there is much disagreement as to radiotherapy's effectiveness—indeed, there have been no conclusive trials. . . . Radiotherapy suffers from the same limitation as surgery, in that it does not affect metastases. . . ."[22]

Dr. Irwin D. J. Bross, director of biostatistics at Roswell Park Memorial Institute, said, "For the situations for which most radiotherapy is given, the chances of curing the patient are probably almost as good as the chances of curing him with laetrile," a substance the doctor appears to have little faith in.[23]

In a study of 3,000 women at 40 institutions, Dr. Bernard Fisher of the University of Pittsburgh found that women receiving radiation following breast cancer surgery showed no higher survival rates than those who received none.[24]

Dr. Israel comments on combined radiation and surgery: "We should observe a reduction in the rate of local recurrences when radiation is added, and no change in the rate of distant metastases . . . in fact, we observe something rather different. Local tumor recurrences . . . do not diminish in cases in which local recurrences are already very rare: a small breast tumor, a peripheral lung tumor. As for distant metastases, certain recent studies have thrown the medical community into confusion by showing that metastases may be more frequent in cases that have received radiation. . . ."[25]

Chemotherapy, like radiotherapy, is highly limited in the number of patients it can actually cure. Like radiation, it often gives fast, temporary relief from tumor growth, thus achieving a reputation as a therapy that cancer "responds" to, but chemotherapy does little good in the long run.

The 30 to 50 poisons used to kill cancer cells are "alkylating agents," which disrupt cell reproduction, "antimetabolites," which prevent cells from making proteins, and "alkaloids," plant-derived poisons.

These poisons offer hope only for some rather rare cancers, and only occasionally prolong life in people with the more common cancers. The cancers that kill most people—breast, colon and lung cancers—generally do not respond to chemotherapy. Chemotherapy is not very effective for any tumor that is large or has spread; its successes are generally with small, very early tumors.[26]

Even temporary cessation of symptoms rarely occurs when chemotherapy is used in cancers of the stomach, bowel, pancreas, cervix and breast. Researcher Victor Richards has found that symptoms from these cancers are lessened "for brief duration in about five to ten per cent of the cases."[27] Richards said in a University of California publication that one of the most valuable roles of chemotherapy is in "keeping the patients oriented toward proper medical therapy and preventing them from the feeling of being abandoned by the physician.[28]

Dr. Israel, who supports use of less strenuous chemotherapeutic programs, says that "the mere word 'chemotherapy' causes an attack of gastric acidity and a sudden rise in blood pressure in many physicians who consider it a dangerous—nay, diabolical—weapon. . . ."[29] Dr. Israel says that many chemotherapies are given in regular, fixed doses, and therefore in gross excess, because of convenience to physicians and because of "intellectual laziness."[30] This results, he says, in frequent failure of the technique.

Chemotherapy, surgery and radiation, the supposedly sophisticated arsenal in our fight against cancer, are, in a sense, outmoded weapons. Trying to use these techniques to cure cancer, said a former N.C.I. head of genetics, is "like trying to put a man on the moon by giving contracts to cannon manufacturers and ladder builders."[31]

Side Effects of the Common Therapies

Simple failure is not the sole problem associated with these three approaches. Their side effects can be ugly and are frequently fatal. Surgery offers the most obvious side effects in its disfigurement, curtailment of function, causing of pain, reduction of immunity, and operative and post-operative death.

Disfigurement can range from scarring, to a loss of breasts or a larynx or limbs, to all-encompassing mutilation. Ralph Moss describes an operation called "total exenteration," which calls for removal of the rectum, stomach, bladder, part of the liver, the ureter, all the internal reproductive organs and pelvic floor and wall, the pancreas, spleen, colon and many of the blood vessels. Its own creator called it "brutal and cruel."[32] Surpassing even this, writes Ralph Moss, is the "hemicorporectomy," or removal of the lower half of the body to "cure" bladder or pelvic malignancy.[33]

Other surgeries also cause suffering. A radical mastectomy can cause lifelong pain. Prostate surgery commonly causes impotence. A hysterectomy causes premature menopause. A laryngectomy causes a loss of one's voice. A colostomy causes loss of control over waste evacuation.

Many surgeries leave patients crippled, debilitated, in pain, or humiliated. Like other of the most common therapies, they are often performed with no hope of achieving recovery.

Surgery depresses immunity, spreads tumors and can cause sudden death. "Most surgeons," two University of Illinois doctors recently told the American Medical Association, "have encountered the patient whose cancer grows rapidly following operation, resulting in death within a few weeks."[34] Surgeries are a great systemic stress, and can cause malignant cells to leave their original site and invade other areas of the body. Many people, of course, die on the operating table, and others die shortly afterward from complications of surgery.

Radiation can cause nausea, and overt weakness and fatigue, sometimes rendering its users bedridden. Excessive fatigue may not sound like a particularly frightening side-effect until one experiences it.

"Radiation," says Dr. Israel," can cause more or less extensive burns of the skin and mucous membranes," and "even very moderate amounts of radiation of the testicles and ovaries may cause sterilization or induce genetic mutations. . . ."[35]

The major problems with radiation are that it severely depresses immunity and can cause chromosome damage resulting in later cancer.

"Radiation," writes Dr. Israel, "can cause a severe and prolonged immune deficiency," not only when it is focused on an organ associated with immunity, such as the thymus, but also when it's focused on areas not associated with immunity. Radiation, he says, "is a two-edged sword. Radiation is carcinogenic at smaller doses than those which immediately injure tissues."[36]

The effects of radiation cancer patients undergo is not substantially different from those suffered by victims of atomic blasts, workers at "leaky" nuclear power facilities, or workers who have to handle uranium. Patients who undergo both chemotherapy and radiation experience later cancers 25 times as often as the general population.[37] The extreme popularity of this doubtful method of disease control gives credence to Dr. Hugh Drummond's dictum on runaway technology: "The history of technology is the history of the invention of hammers and the subsequent search for heads to bang them with."[38]

Chemotherapy is noted for the symptoms of nausea it causes, the death from toxicity it causes, its depression of immunity, and the fact that it can be carcinogenic.

Chemotherapy exerts particularly strong poisonous effects upon cells in the gut and hair follicles, causing extreme nausea and vomiting, baldness, bleeding gums, sores around the mouth, and bleeding and ulceration of the gastrointestinal tract. Chemotherapy's side effects have been said by many cancer patients to be more unpleasant than the pain of the disease.

Patients undergoing chemotherapy suffer extremely depressed immunity, and have been known to die from minor infections, or even colds. "Chemotherapy," writes Ralph Moss, "often brings in its train a host of blood-deficiency diseases, such as leukopenia, thrombocytopenia and aplastic anemia."[39]

One study indicated that as many as 10 to 20 per cent of all patients undergoing chemotherapy die directly from the toxic effects of the drugs upon their weakened systems. A study reported in the *New York State Journal of Medicine* of 133 patients, all using the chemotherapeutic agent 5-FU, showed that 10 per cent of these patients died as a direct result of 5-FU toxicity.[40]

If these common therapies are indeed associated with many problems, why, many people ask, do they predominate as the major therapies for cancer?

The Common Therapies' Support Systems

These therapies have two primary systems supporting them, an economic one and a philosophical one.

Obviously, these drug and technological approaches are profitable, and therefore have a built-in rationale for existence. Chemotherapy is a $200 million per year business, and stock analysts say that it will someday do a billion dollars worth of business per year.[41] "Drugs are central to the American economy," writes Moss, "and it is perfectly logical from a business point of view to seek a cure for cancer in the form of a patentable, marketable drug."[42]

Radiation is a high-profit venture, and one that requires a considerable outlay of venture capital. A hospital can easily spend up to $5 million in modernizing its radiology department. Obviously, this sort of investment must be taken advantage of by frequent use of the purchased equipment.

Surgery, likewise, tends sometimes to be dictated as much by its availability as by its need. Countries with fewer surgeons commonly experience markedly fewer unnecessary surgeries. Surgeries, also, are paid for on a "piecework" basis. As George Bernard Shaw once pointed out, "The more appalling the mutilation, the more the mutilator is paid." Most surgeons, of course, do not coldly plot unnecessary operations—their motivation to over-use the scalpel stems from far more subtle feelings, and, in many cases, doubtless stems from a genuine desire to help.

The philosophical bias toward these approaches hinges on a faith in mechanistic medicine's technology, a vision of the doctor as a superman, and a lack of reliance upon personal immune strength. These same traits characterize many aspects of what we identify as modern medicine.

The attitude many mechanistic cancer therapists approach their work with is, finally, somewhat of an extension of the military mind-frame. This "macho medical militancy," says medical writer Peter Barry Chowka, presumes that the "war on cancer" can be won if enough firepower is brought to bear on the situation. One invasive surgery of the jaw is called the "commando" operation, because, according to Dr. George Crile, "it brought to mind the slashing attack of the World War commandos."[43] Radiation against cancer is frequently equated with radiation-based bombs. "Atomic medicine," says the *New York Times,* "focuses the powerful beams of deadly rays."[44] The question invariably posed about new chemotherapy agents is: "Will this be the 'magic bullet'?"

It is a shame that this "invasive mentality," with its disdain for the strength of the human immune response, is so prevalent. This is very sad, because, without doubt, simple human immune response probably offers the best answer to cancer. Most cancer patients go to their graves having never been allowed to know this.

PART THREE

The Metabolic Approach to Cancer

Above all, it frightens me that everything I am saying has already been said.

—Jacobo Timermal

CHAPTER NINE

The Metabolic Approach to Cancer

There is nothing particularly magical about the metabolic approach to cancer. It is not a drug or chemical "magic bullet." It does not use the "magic wand" of technological gimmickry. It does not depend upon the magical ministrations of the attending physician. Actually, nothing could be more down-to-earth than the common sense advice that composes this approach.

This approach, advocated by Dr. W. D. Kelley and the physicians with whom he consults, is simply health stimulation carried out systematically.

Out of respect for the marvels of the human body, doctors who administer metabolic therapy readily admit that they aren't even aware of all the ways that the body reverses cancer during application of this approach. It was not even known until the latter 1970s, for example, that certain white blood cells "spotted and marked" cancer cells, in preparation for invasion by "killer" white blood cells. Likewise, the medical community still doesn't know, and may never know, every exact function of the liver. There are undoubtedly anti-cancer liver functions that are yet to be catalogued. Therefore, metabolic doctors bow to the innate "knowledge" held by the body, and support the body with common sense measures. They don't pretend to be omnipotently directing every anti-malignant function that takes place.

The metabolic approach affects a multitude of conditions other than malignancy. Metabolic therapy is effective in countering malignancy, but is also effective in other ways. It is a "non-specific therapy," a therapy that helps the body to rid itself of many different diseases and to achieve a state of optimum health. Each person's metabolic program is different, because of individual differences in metabolism and lifestyle, and because of existence of different diseases.

Hundreds of doctors in America employ the metabolic approach: they attempt to solve health problems by stimulating the patient's entire energy exchange with the environment, or "metabolism." No formal State Board Certification currently exists for metabolic doctors, just as, for example, there is no current state certification for the allergy-related medical doctors who practice as "clinical ecologists." Therefore, the term is often used rather loosely, by a large number of professionally unrelated physicians.

Many of these physicians attend the seminars, sponsored by Dr. Kelley, and regularly consult with him. People who wish to contact any of these doctors may call the International Health Institute, a non-profit Dallas, Texas, informational agency which assists people in finding the type of professional help that they feel they need.

Cover All Your Bases

The metabolic approach has three mechanisms that work against cancer cells. One is specifically anti-tumoral. An example of this facet is use of high doses of enzymes, which appear to directly attack the cancer cell walls. Another mechanism is the stimulation of the immune system. This facet includes use of vitamins A and C, which bolster natural immunity. The third mechanism is health stimulation of the entire system. An example of this is the positive-thinking aspect of the approach, which seems to help the body conquer cancer, but also helps the rest of the system deal with any problems that may be present.

It is considered very important to create programs that are individualized. Until just the past few years, the rarely-questioned goal of almost every medical therapy was to make the therapy work equally well upon every person. Therapies had to be fully "replicable" in person after person to be considered valid. This is still, in many circles, a much-vaunted criterion of validity. But this notion of all humans responding with unvarying similarity to identical treatments goes against the grain of good sense. All people were created un-equally; our Creator did not stamp us all out with the same cookie-cutter. We were not rendered indistinguishable from one another in biochemistry, structure, and genetic and emotional makeup. We are all so vastly different that to apply the same therapy to every person guarantees failure in a great many cases. An approach that works well for a vegetarian-oriented young woman with no major stresses in her life might be an absolute disaster for a middle-aged, meat-eating man who runs a complex business.

The metabolic approach to cancer is based on evidence that many factors are involved in cancer causation and that a multi-faceted health program is needed to defeat cancer. Based on many years of clinical observation and study of the literature, metabolic researchers now believe that every disease, including cancer, is the result of a number of negative influences upon health, and that a collection of positive influences must therefore be a part of every healing program. Colon cancer, for example, is thought to begin to form because of too much fat and not enough fiber in the diet, which creates the toxic condition of excessive bile acid secretion. The colon cancer may then be promoted by a lack of certain vitamins that normally deactivate bile alkaloids, an exhausted liver that has been over-used to compensate for toxicity, and the generally debilitating effects of the stress of a fast-paced, tiring lifestyle. This is actually a gross simplification of the multi-faceted nature of cancer causation. In reality, as many as 50 or more factors may combine to disrupt the normal bodily processes. Cancer, of course, is just one possible outcome of these health insults.

It seems to metabolic doctors to be patently unintelligent, a model of naivete, to think that any single therapeutic agent, whether it is radiation or vitamin C or emotional counseling, will reverse this complex condition. Any single-factor therapy, they believe, is almost certain to fail to repair all the weak and broken links in this ruptured chain of health. Radiation may temporarily shrink a tumor in the colon, but will it repair an ulcerated colon wall? Vitamin C may help the immune system to kill tumor cells, but will it improve the body with the nutrients it needs to repair ravaged tissue? These rhetorical questions point to a principle considered of vital importance by metabolic physicians: Cover all your bases.

A multi-faceted approach, say metabolic doctors, helps each organ. A colon attacked by malignancy may need a special diet, but may also need increased detoxification, as well as a relaxation of emotion-caused muscular tension. Each organ needs a variety of help.

The organ that is under direct attack, though, is not the only organ that needs help. No organ is an island unto itself. All organs and systems are dependent upon one another. How ridiculous it is, for example, to try to improve the function of the large intestine without trying to help the small intestine! The very words we use to describe our body's physical components—organs and systems—connote interdependence. The whole crux of the "holistic" healing philosophy is to treat the whole body, rather than just isolated parts of it—if, indeed, there are "isolated" parts of the body. The head bone is, as they say, connected to the neck bone.

The goal of metabolic physicians, therefore, is to use many methods to improve the function of many glands, organs and systems. This "cover-all-your-bases" approach promotes an extraordinary, synergistic chain reaction of healing. Every system in the body is improved by every aspect of the program, and each system, in turn, helps improve the function of every other system. Thus, a downward spiral of degeneration is transformed into an upward spiral of regeneration.

Computer Age Medicine

The various aspects of each person's individualized program can be compiled by use of computer-evaluated questionnaires and blood and urine testing. This testing is done by metabolic physicians at the same time that disease risk factors and immune strength are evaluated by the patient evaluation procedure.

This type of computer evaluation is done by asking clients many questions about disease risk-factors, health history, dietary and health habits, physical and emotional condition, etc. Results of information given the computer can be cross-checked against other information given it, in order to insure accuracy of responses.

A properly devised evaluative process can assess many different health indices, including efficiency of vitamin and mineral metabolism, amounts of various nutrients in the blood, level of function of all major organs, systems and glands, state of emotional and spiritual strength, efficiency of hormonal and enzymatic activity, possible structural abnormalities, presence of toxins, etc. Extrapolating from this information, trained physicians can note proneness to cancer and other diseases.

Based upon this type of evaluation, a proper, individualized program can be created. This program can help to stimulate optimum health, and to assist the body in reversing any pathologies, including cancer, which may be present.

The metabolic approach basically consists of six components. They are: (1) diet, (2) food supplementation, (3) detoxification, (4) structural therapy, (5) emotional therapy, and (6) lifestyle change. These aspects compose the basis of the proper metabolic anti-cancer programs.

Diet

Dietary considerations of key importance are: the individualization of diets; the use of diets to provide enhanced nutrition; the use of diets to help detoxify the gastrointestinal tract, organs of elimination and other cells throughout the body; and the use of diets to help balance the nervous system.

Some patients naturally thrive on diets high in complex proteins, particularly meat, while others are unable to readily digest meat and other high-protein foods. If people eat diets that are contrary to their own biochemical and metabolic needs, they gradually become quite prone to a degenerative disease. Other factors that create a need for individualized diets include presence of allergic reaction to foods, condition of the nervous system, the demands of one's lifestyle, and one's genetic heritage.

Most people with cancer appear to need a vegetarian-oriented diet early in their therapy, because they need to divert protein-digesting pancreatic enzymes to their tumors; the enzymes, as we've stated, are thought to help break down cancer cell walls. A vegetarian diet is very easy to digest, which relieves stress upon the liver, pancreas, gall bladder, stomach and intestines. It provides a maximum of vitamins, minerals and enzymes. People whose biochemistries are oriented toward vegetarianism remain on this diet indefinitely, while natural carnivores move gradually to high-protein diets as their malignancies recede.

Maximum nutrition must be gleaned from one's diet in order to nourish the immune system, to help repair damaged tissue, to stimulate the vital organs, and to maintain adequate physical and mental strength during the ordeal of illness. Some of these badly-needed nutrients, such as vitamins C and A, stimulate immune function. Others, such as enzymes found in foods, seem to have direct anti-tumoral effects. Enzymes and certain vitamins can neutralize toxic agents in the bloodstream that come from the malignant tumor. All nutrients are important in rebuilding damaged tissues and organs, and helping these tissues and organs resist the onslaught of future malignancy. This protection and repair is of crucial importance, since tissue and organ damage is frequently the cause of death during cancer. It is also important in that cancer cannot be defeated by the body's own recuperative systems unless those systems are functioning adequately.

Dietary considerations can be used to help rebalance the "autonomic nervous system," the part of the nervous system that controls involuntary acts, including all those activities associated with metabolism. Most people with a serious disease, say metabolic doctors, tend to have an autonomic nervous system that is excessively shifted toward either its "speed-up" (sympathetic) branch, or its "slow-down" (parasympathetic) branch. This causes glandular and organ malfunction. A vegetarian-oriented diet, because of its effects on the brain's nerve transmission, tends to promote stimulation of the parasympathetic branch. Stimulating this branch seems to be most helpful for diminishing tumors; the reasons for this are discussed in the following chapter.

All diets should be based on pure, whole foods, with minimal additives. These foods provide maximum nutrition and ease of digestion, and minimal toxicity.

For details, see the chapter "The Anti-Cancer Diet."

Food Supplementation

Food supplementation, strictly speaking, is a facet of diet, though many people tend to think of supplements as medicine. In a sense, supplements are medicine: Hippocrates said, "Let food be your medicine and let medicine be your food."

Supplements are concentrated nutrients. In most of our food today, because of hybridization, depleted soils, and artificial stimulation of growth, it is quite difficult to find sufficient nutrients. It is almost impossible for anyone with cancer to receive the high amounts of nutrients needed to overcome the disease without supplementation.

People with cancer are advised by metabolic doctors to take high doses of many vitamins, minerals, enzymes and glandular extracts. Vitamins, minerals, enzymes and other supplements appear to be tumor-specific, tissue reparative, immune stimulative, can detoxify, can stimulate organ and glandular function, and can help regulate neurological function.

Glandular extracts, tissues taken directly from the glands of animals, have been proven by radioimmunoassay tests to travel directly to the corresponding gland of the person ingesting the extract, supplying the person's gland with the specific amino acids and other nutrients needed, and stimulating the gland to increased activity. Extracts from glands and organs associated with immunity and resistance to cancer, such as thymus and liver extract, are considered to be of special value for cancer patients. Glandulars can also help influence the nervous system. Stimulation, for example, of the anterior medial hypothalamus, thymus, stomach, liver, pancreas, spleen and adrenal cortex, can shift a patient toward the "healing" condition of parasympathetic dominance.

People seem to do best when they take concentrated whole-food nutrients, rather than synthetically derived vitamins or minerals, because there are many important substances in foods that have not yet been identified, extracted and concentrated by nutritional scientists. These substances are not only valuable in themselves, but also exert a catalytic effect upon other nutrients.

For details, see the chapter on anti-cancer supplementation.

Detoxification

Metabolic doctors do not consider it sufficient to merely deactivate cancer cells, toxic agents and harmful cellular material—these substances must also be eliminated from the body. The neutralizing of harmful chemicals, which occurs naturally and can be aided by nutrients, such as vitamins C and A and certain enzymes, is sometimes also considered a facet of detoxification.

Flushing destructive materials from the body is a constant, ongoing function. Elimination occurs through the kidneys, liver, colon, skin and lungs. Facilitating this process is of great importance to cancer patients, who kill so many cells every day, once their metabolic therapy starts, that they are in danger of suffering severe toxic reaction, and even death, from a back-up of elimination. If the organs of elimination cannot accept further toxic materials, these materials will remain in the circulatory and lymphatic systems and may return to the cells.

The only unpleasant side effect of a metabolic program for cancer patients, and for other people who are consciously creating a rapid cell turnover, is a feeling of being "toxic," which results from killing more cells than can be eliminated from the system. The experience feels somewhat like having the flu. To relieve and prevent this feeling, it is helpful to stimulate rapid elimination of toxic agents, or "detoxify" the body. This can be done with coffee enemas, liver and gall bladder flushes, controlled sweating, detoxification baths, exercise, dry skin brushing and stimulation of the kidneys with diuretics and juices.

Coffee enemas, introduced to cancer patients by Max Gerson, M.D., in the 1940s, are a powerful stimulant to the liver. The caffeine from the coffee travels through the portal vein directly into the liver, greatly stimulating its function. There have been attempts of late by some members of the medical community to assert that this simple healing technique poses some biochemical hazard. Literally every single practitioner who recommends the procedure, however, has reported that it is safe and effective; adverse reactions are virtually unheard of among active users of the technique. On the contrary, most people report that the coffee enema, done daily or several times weekly, improves their general feeling of well-being, negates toxicity, and improves mood and energy. The amount of caffeine absorbed into the system is slight; almost all is absorbed by the liver or excreted with the coffee.

Liver and gall bladder purges, done with the traditional use of olive oil and lemon juice, are quite valuable in the non-surgical removal of gallstones, solid debris and bile from these organs. It is recommended that this procedure be done by cancer patients almost once a month, since the liver function of cancer patients is generally impaired. Most patients report a surge of well-being following the procedure.

Stimulating the egress of toxins through the urine and perspiration is also valuable, and is easily and safely done. Saunas and dry skin brushing clean the epidermis, open pores and stimulate sweating. Herbal diuretics and fruit juices are helpful in stimulating the kidneys. Rapid dispelling of toxins through the kidneys and skin relieves the burden on the over-worked liver of the cancer patient.

Detoxification is often as pleasant as it is therapeutic. Many people report feeling better after some of the procedures.

For details, see the chapter on detoxification and cancer.

Structural Therapy

Structural (skeletal) problems can, according to metabolic doctors, cause biochemical abnormalities that result in malignancies, and sometimes structural problems are a result of malignancy or disrupted biochemistry. In either case, they can "lock in" pathology, making biochemical intervention difficult or even almost impossible. Impingement upon the tenth cranial nerve, which supplies the stomach, pancreas, liver, lungs and heart, is frequently considered to be a contributing factor to malignancy. This impingement, which most often occurs as the nerve passes by the "temporomandibular joint" in the jaw, can be mediated by a structural therapy called "mandibular equilibration." Other forms of structural therapy that are often considered of vital importance to the cancer patient are chiropractic, cranial osteopathy, spinal column stressology (a whole-spine therapy), reflexology (a form of massage based on acupuncture points) and Swedish massage. Any impairment of nerve function to a vital organ or gland may be sufficient to tip the balance of a patient's health toward the range of pathology, and may be enough to render even the best nutritional therapy insufficient.

Structural problems are often overlooked by even presumably "holistic" practitioners, in defiance of a basic law of physics, which metabolic doctors believe applies to humans: "Function follows form." Bodies that are in continual neurological disorder are not usually biochemically balanced, and bodies under the constant stress of misalignment are being chronically drained of energy. A person with cancer, whose health is already being taxed, cannot tolerate this extra stress.

For details, see the chapter on structural therapy and cancer.

Emotional Therapy

Emotional problems have been shown by Dr. O. Carl Simonton, Dr. Lawrence LeShan and others to be significant contributing factors to malignancy. Internalized conflict, belief systems characterized by helplessness and hopelessness, and a spiritual attitude of living a senseless, terminal existence are all considered to be part of the "carcinogenic personality." Cancer patients' mental problems often are manifested as physical problems, either because of unhealthy lifestyles that are a result of emotional turmoil, or because of direct impairment of vital systems, including the immune system, by stress-related factors. People with cancer who do not address the psychological components of their disease are said to often have incredible difficulty in instituting necessary healing changes into their lifestyles.

People often make remarkable recoveries from cancer after thay have overcome emotional problems, which often include emotional rigidity, feelings of guilt and inadequacy, and submerged anger. People with cancer should be encouraged to discharge their feelings, to reassert their will to live, to relax, to enjoy life, and to think positively. If they can achieve these things, they often experience a resurgence of the recuperative powers of the body.

No researcher at this point is exactly sure how the emotions and systems of immunity are connected, but virtually the entire medical community now accepts the fact that there is indeed a link.

Emotions must be dealt with differently for each patient. A properly systematized patient evaluation procedure can determine if people need emotional help, but they are allowed to select the kind of help they feel most comfortable with.

Similarly, spiritual unease is thought to sometimes be a significant factor in diseases, including cancer. A feeling of alienation from the rest of the world, a lack of a code of moral values, and a sense of life's finiteness all seem to have a strong negative impact upon a person's survival possibilities. People who have faith in religion or who have a firm belief system appear to fare much better. People should try to reconcile their spiritual attitudes; when they do this, doctors often find that their health improves. No one really knows why this happens, but it does appear to occur regularly.

For details, see the chapter on the emotional and spiritual aspects of cancer.

Lifestyle Change

Lifestyle changes—involving increased rest, relaxation, exercise, and limitation of exposure to carcinogenic substances—differ with each person. Generally, people are advised to minimize stressful factors and curtail as much as possible further health insults to their bodies. Exercise is considered to be of special benefit in improving oxygenation of cells, which is specifically helpful for cancer patients, and for inducing muscular and emotional relaxation. Almost all people with cancer should purify their personal living situations as much as possible, in order to focus the detoxification and immune processes on elimination of existing toxins in the body.

Lifestyle change, of course, is a very personal endeavor. Areas that seem to be in need of change can be determined through the evaluative process with the patient, but the refining and instituting of these changes is, by necessity, a matter of personal responsibility.

For details, see the chapter "The Anti-Cancer Lifestyle."

Health Doesn't Hurt!

Health programs are often rigorous, but they are not painful. In fact, once people become accustomed to integrating these habits into their lives, and once they become familiar with the exhilaration that generally accompanies these health-promoting habits, it is almost impossible for most of them to go back to the self-destructive patterns that contributed to the causation of their disease.

These health programs require only perseverance, moderation, and a little discipline. This is a paltry fee, indeed, to pay for freedom from a disease so insidious as cancer.

CHAPTER TEN

Individualizing the Anti-Cancer Program

Two primary concepts considered absolutely necessary for a superior metabolic program are: (1) the non-specific concept, which calls for addressing all aspects of all parts of the body, and (2) the concept of metabolic individuality, which says that every person is different and must be dealt with differently.

Application of the principle of metabolic individuality is considered absolutely imperative in helping people with cancer recover. The principle of individuality, according to metabolic doctors, must be implemented in conjunction with that of non-specificity, which is to say, simply, that patients must be treated individualistically in all of the components of their health. These components include nutrition, supplementation, structure, detoxification, emotions, and lifestyle habits.

A lack of appreciation for individualization is rampant in the technological medical community, because of that community's infatuation with the replicability and interchangeability of therapies. The highest goal for most medical therapies is that the identical procedure or drug work equally well on all patients, regardless of the differences in patients. This goal fits superbly with the technological-medicine concept that all humans are essentially similar, albeit complicated, biomechanical machines. The belief that we all rolled off the same assembly line gives credence to treating us all with similar chemicals, and replacing our "broken parts" with plastic "organs" and "bones" and "ligaments."

This concept of sameness, though, is not in accord with reality, and successes derived from it are almost often successes of symptom-suppression, rather than restoration of health. For example, digitalis may well seem to improve the cardiovascular function of three different people, one with hardened arteries, one with fat-clogged arteries, and one with an atrophied heart muscle. However, metabolic doctors believe that only three different therapy programs, composed of detoxification, nutrition, supplementation, exercise and lifestyle change, will actually alter the conditions of all three patients. If, by the same token, all three engaged in one standardized, rigid health program, quite possibly none would recover.

A lack of appreciation of individuality is also, in the opinion of the authors of this book, frequently found in the therapies of supposedly holistic doctors. This lack of appreciation is a major failing of many physicians practicing presumably holistic cancer therapy. A simplistic natural cancer therapy, such as the one called the "Grape Cure," may work for a few people, including those who thrive on a basically fruitarian diet and who are in severe need of a powerful detoxifying diet, but it will fail for most people. All of the essentially vegetarian-diet cancer therapies, such as the Hippocrates Health Institute's wheatgrass-oriented therapy, will work well for people who naturally thrive on vegetarian diets. These therapies, though, do not appear to us to be equally effective for cancer patients who are natural carnivores, as many Americans are. Likewise, most of the therapies centered around laetrile seem to get good results in a certain number of patients, but are far too standardized in their healing programs. Dwight McKee, M.D., recently observed the work being done at several laetrile clinics and reported, "Too many of the physicians are still working within outmoded philosophical confines. They're operating under the misconception that each approach or substance has to work the same for everyone or it's not predictable, and therefore unreliable, and therefore worthless. Standardization is an outdated concept that they still believe in.

"Some of these supposedly progressive clinics," says Dr. McKee, "are identical to the mechanical-medical model. The patients eat a standardized diet, line up for injections of vitamins and enzymes, and go through the same therapeutic regimes, all together, under some authority's direction."

There Is No Human Assembly Line

However much mankind wishes to be a collection of simple machines with interchangeable parts, the wish will never be granted.

Roger Williams, Ph.D., of the University of Texas, has devoted a lifetime to proving the importance of treating patients individualistically. Dr. Williams writes, "Everyone accepts the fact that each person's fingerprints are unique, yet few realize that inborn individuality extends beyond the whorls on a person's fingertips; it pervades every part of the body. From birth, human beings are highly distinctive in both microscopic and gross anatomy, in functioning of their organs, the composition of body fluids, and in their nutritional requirements.

"Barry Anson of Northwestern University was the first anatomist to stress the widespread differences in the anatomy of "normal" human beings. His *Atlas of Human Anatomy* shows remarkable variations in normal human stomachs, livers, nerves, and muscles and in the branching of the arteries in the aortic arch, a portion of the main artery that rises from the heart's left ventricle. About 65 per cent of people have three arteries branching off the aorta; this is considered the normal arrangement. But about 35 per cent have, instead of three branches, one, two, four, five or six.

"If the aortic arch is typical of human variation (and studies suggest that it is), it is likely that practically every human being is atypical in some respects. W. Duane Brown provided support for this theory when he analyzed blood samples taken from 11 healthy young men. Once a week for five to six weeks, he collected a blood sample from each man after the volunteers had fasted. When Brown compared the levels of different constituents in the volunteers' blood with the composition of supposedly normal blood, he found that each man's blood was unique. No individual's blood corresponded in all respects to normal blood, nor was any volunteer's blood exactly like that of another.

"Disparities like those found by Anson and Brown exist in all the structures of the human body as well as in the constituents of all body fluids. According to Anson, some anatomical features have been depicted as normal in medical books for generations, yet they probably apply to only 15 per cent of the population.

"These differences are permanent—one obviously does not have one arrangement of arteries or muscles at one stage in life and some other arrangement at other times—and they are genetically determined. The influence of heredity also extends to the structure and metabolism of every cell. It is well established that genes determine the speed and efficiency with which cells perform their essential functions.

"The fact that every newborn infant has a distinctive physical makeup has a profound influence on every person's future. First, it makes a definition of "normal" impossible. Second, it means that our individuality exists before external influences can affect us, and that unless the environment can satisfy at least our most basic genetically programmed needs, we will die."[1]

Nutritional Individuality

Dr. Williams believes that meeting the differing nutritional needs of individuals is the most important single aspect in the individualization of health care. Individualization of diet is possibly no more important than individualization of, for example, emotional or structural therapy, but the emotional and structural aspects of health tend to be naturally met with an individualized therapy. Nutrition, though, is quite often approached with the old-fashioned "blanket approach."

The history of the concept of nutritional individuality is not a lengthy one.

Dr. George Watson, of the University of Southern California, was one of the first men to acknowledge that there were, indeed, different types of metabolisms, or energy exchanges with the environment. Dr. Watson noted in the 1960s that different foods have drastic effects on the emotions of different people, depending on whether they are fast or slow burners of food, or "oxidizers." Fast oxidizers, he noted, need slow-to-digest food in order to keep their blood sugar and hormone levels stable and to avoid drastic mood fluctuations. Slow oxidizers, though, become overtly sluggish if they eat more food than they can metabolize.

Dr. Watson was struck by the relative ease of eliminating neurotic and psychotic symptoms by altering nutritional patterns. He noted that the rather arbitrarily manufactured "minimum daily requirements" of vitamins and minerals are applicable only to "average" people, and that a huge per cent of all people are not at all average in their biochemical needs. He was among the first to draw the distinction between "minimum" nutritional requirements and "optimum" requirements. Dr. Watson found that many patients' emotional health improved infinitely when they shifted from minimum to optimum levels of nutrients.[2]

Concurrent with the work of Dr. Watson was that of Dr. Williams, who has long championed the concept of nutritional individuality. Dr. Williams, in his book *Biochemical Individuality,* advanced the "genetotrophic" principle—the idea that all people are genetically predisposed to have specific biochemical needs, which must be met with the proper nutrients. Dr. Williams believes that virtually all degenerative disease, including cancer, is caused by "cellular malnutrition,"[4] and can be prevented and sometimes corrected by ending this malnutrition. Cancer is currently epidemic, eventually striking one out of four people, he believes, primarily because of the generally deplorable food consumed in highly industrialized societies, which affords little if any margin for variances in individualized needs. This view of biochemical deficiency and imbalance as a major contributor to chronic, degenerative disease is shared by almost all metabolic, holistic practitioners.

Dr. Williams, the first biochemist to be elected president of the American Chemical Society and the discoverer of pantothenic acid, wrote in *Nutrition Against Disease,* "That malnutrition—unbalanced or inadequate nutrition—at the cellular level, should be thought of as a major cause of human disease seems crystal clear to me. It is the inevitable conclusion to be drawn from the facts produced by decades of biochemical research.

"What do these facts suggest in terms of practical application? We need to develop techniques for identifying far more accurately than is now possible the inherited pattern of susceptibilities and resistances that is unique to each individual.

Call it a 'metabolic profile' or any other name you wish, but plainly it represents a necessary precondition for making rational programs of nutrition tailored to fit each individual's special requirements."[3]

Making Individuality Work for You

Dr. Williams created a strong theoretical foundation for nutritional individuality, but did not apply his work to patients. The first efforts to make the concept available for use with patients were those of physicians working with the computerized health information gathered by Dr. W. D. Kelley.

Various doctors had been doing metabolic rebalancing before the advent of the nutritional individuality concept. Their programs were quite successful for many people suffering from cancer, heart disease, arthritis, multiple sclerosis, diabetes and a host of other degenerative ailments. But they weren't successful for all people.

After Dr. Kelley had recovered from metastasized liver-pancreatic cancer, he was enthusiastic about the metabolic program he'd followed—a vegetarian diet, supplements and detoxification. Since he had been so successful, he mistakenly thought his program would work on everybody.

To deal with her own serious health problems, his wife embarked upon a diet and supplementation program similar to his. Disaster ensued. She developed strong allergies, intense depression and energy loss so severe that she lapsed in and out of a three-week coma. She improved dramatically when her diet and supplementation were restructured, by trial and error, to fit her own particular metabolism.

It was through this experience that Dr. Kelley began to reformulate his ideas. He began listening intently to people who would say that certain vitamins, minerals and foods made them feel better or worse. He corroborated these reported responses with metabolic testing procedures. Some supplements and foods worked well for some people, while the same supplements and foods caused other people to feel terrible. From close observation and from reports from physicians of clinical experiences with many disease conditions, he began to classify people into different types.

He devised a numerical scale, with the slow-oxidizing vegetarians at one extreme and the fast-oxidizing carnivores at the other extreme. By classifying each person into his or her own proper type, it made it easier to determine what vitamins, minerals, foods and other supplements would best enhance each person's own body chemistry. Even more importantly, it became possible to quickly tell what supplements and foods people should not have. By proper classification of each individual, it saved physicians the long, tedious trial and error of experimentation with each of their patients.

Computerized Nutritional Therapy

Dr. Kelley realized that not many people could come in person to be individually tested. If this concept were ever to be in widespread use, it would have to be in a form that local doctors and lay metabolic technicians could use.

Because of this need, he created a patient evaluation procedure. The procedure, which evaluates one's health, includes as part of its evaluative process an indication of what a person's "metabolic type" is, as well as one's "sub-type" (the category other than one's type that one has the most tendencies toward), and one's "developmental type" (the type one was as a child).

Dr. Kelley discovered that a person's metabolic type, which he now considers information essential in helping a person recover from cancer, is determined by more than whether or not the person is oriented toward a vegetarian or carnivorous diet. The most important aspect determining nutritional individuality rests, he found, in the nervous system.

The Key to Metabolism

The body has two nervous systems—the central, which governs conscious movement, and the autonomic, governing unconscious actions like digestion, secretion, breathing and heartbeat. The autonomic nervous system is the master regulator of metabolism, including metabolism at the cellular level. It determines how outside sources of energy, such as food, water, light, temperature, etc., are going to be used to support life, and how efficiently these sources of energy are going to be used.

The autonomic nervous system has two branches. Both of them—the sympathetic and parasympathetic—send electric impulses to all our glands, organs and systems. The sympathetic's basic message is "speed up," the parasympathetic's is "slow down." Most people, we believe, because of their genetic makeup, and structural and nutritional factors, have a relatively more active sympathetic or parasympathetic branch. This facet of their physical makeup is of the utmost importance in determining metabolic tendencies, such as the rate of oxidation.

The rate of oxidation, of course, determines whether one needs fast-burning or slow-burning food, and when one needs to be eating it. A fast-oxidizer, obviously, will grow hungry and weak between meals of fast-burning food. Various glands, organs and systems in the body, including the immune system, decrease or increase in activity during these energy lulls. A slow-oxidizer will thrive on easily digested, high carbohydrate, low-protein foods, and will cause himself or herself health problems by eating food that is difficult to digest, such as fatty meat.

Metabolism involves far more factors, though, than merely rate of oxidation. Sympathetic or parasympathetic dominance plays a part in innumerable other biological actions.

Glandular and organ function is governed by the autonomic nervous system. People with sympathetic dominance seem to have abundant nerve stimulation to the adrenal medulla, posterior lateral hypothalamus, anterior pituitary, pineal, thyroid, parathyroid and gonads. Parasympathetic dominant people seem to have strong nerve stimulation to the anterior medial hypothalamus, posterior pituitary, thymus, stomach, pancreas, liver, spleen, intestinal tract and adrenal cortex. The various activities of these glands and organs are associated with resistance or susceptibility to various diseases. For example, research has shown that proper functioning of the thymus, pancreas and liver, and adequate hydrochloric acid secretion in the stomach, are all linked to cancer immunity. Many researchers who believe the immune system is the major factor in cancer resistance have acknowledged that these organs and glands, which tend to function well in parasympathetic dominant people, are of primary importance in cancer immunity. As a consequence, a majority of those who contract cancer seem to be sympathetic dominant. This also explains why a vegetarian diet with the appropriate supplements is—for sympathetic dominant people with cancer—a good form of nutritional therapy.

Dominance of the two branches of the autonomic nervous system is also associated with basic energy levels, moods and biochemical balances. A sympathetic dominant person, for example, besides being a slow-metabolizing person who does well on a vegetarian-oriented diet, tends to be energetic, and more acid in body chemistry than alkaline. A parasympathetic dominant person, a fast-oxidizer who needs meat, tends to be more lethargic, prone to allergies and depression, and more alkaline than acid. These traits stem from the nerve stimulation that various glands and organs receive. The sympathetic dominant person's high energy, for instance, is tied to the stimulation of the energy-boosting adrenal medulla, while the parasympathetic dominant person's fast digestion is owed to stimulation of the stomach, pancreas and intestinal tract.

It appears to metabolic doctors as if various disease states tend to accompany sympathetic or parasympathetic dominance. Sympathetic dominant people are prone to bacterial infections, diabetes, ulcerative colitis, rheumatoid arthritis, arteriosclerosis, cancer, acne, and hypertension. Parasympathetics are prone to asthma, low blood pressure, hypoglycemia, edema, leukemia, lymphoma, melanoma, Hodgkin's disease, viral infections and mucous colitis. Each of these disorders is associated with the function of different organs and glands, and with biochemical conditions which are influenced by stimulation from the autonomic nervous system.

Psychological traits associated with sympathetic dominance are ambition and drive, frequent mood swings, a quick temper, a preference for high levels of activity and decision-making, strongly felt emotions, and a tendency toward increased sexuality. These mental and emotional traits are linked to the sympathetic dominant person's slow oxidizing, with the elevated stimulation of the adrenal medulla, with the increased function of hormone-producing glands such as the gonads, and with the generalized "accelerator" function of the sympathetic nervous system.

Parasympathetic dominant people, on the other hand, tend to be more calm, less energetic and ambitious, and have a tendency toward depression. These traits are linked to increased nerve activity to the adrenal cortex, which exerts a "braking" action, with the generalized "decelerator" function of the parasympathetic nervous system, and with the relatively reduced activity of the areas of the brain that secrete the neurotransmitters dopamine, epinephrine and norepinephrine, which are associated with feelings of happiness and well-being.

Altering the Imbalance

Neither parasympathetic nor sympathetic dominance is preferable. Each has, in physical and emotional manifestations, its benefits and drawbacks. There is, however, a desired condition: balance. It appears as if people with finely balanced nervous systems tend to have balanced biochemistries, emotional stability, and strong immune resistance to cancer. A person with a highly-charged sympathetic nervous system and a minimally functioning parasympathetic nervous system will be quite vulnerable to the health problems associated with strong sympathetic dominance. People with very dominant sympathetic nervous systems seem quite vulnerable to cancer. After determining the branch predominance and degree of predominance of the autonomic nervous system with the patient evaluation procedure, we try to balance the autonomic nervous system as much as possible. If either branch of the autonomic nervous system is allowed to predominate unduly, the organs and glands stimulated by that branch may function so strenuously that they "overpower" the organs and glands of the opposite branch, causing deleterious biochemical imbalances. If this situation continues for months or years, these overstimulated organs and glands may become taxed to the point of exhaustion and malfunction. Imbalance, in fact, is a common condition, and it is often one of the major predisposing factors to degenerative diseases, including cancer.

The situation, however, can be remedied. Metabolic type, determined by heredity, structural factors and nutritional factors, can be influenced by structural and nutritional manipulation.

One can't, of course, alter one's heredity. If a person has a genetic background strongly based in ancestors who lived in tropical or semitropical areas and who ate primarily fruits and vegetables, one will be predisposed toward a vegetarian, sympathetic-dominant metabolism. If most or all of one's ancestors were cold-climate consumers of high protein animal products, one will be more likely to have a parasympathetic, meat-eating metabolism.

An example of a structural factor that can influence metabolic type is impingement by the cranial bones on the vagus nerve, which supplies most of the nerve stimulation to the digestive organs. If this impairment exists, the parasympathetic nervous system will suffer, and an imbalance is very likely to occur. Several techniques can remedy problems like this, including cranial osteopathy, mandibular equilibration, spinal column stressology, and cranial chiropractic.

Nutrition is the easiest and often most effective way to influence one's metabolic type. It can be used in strict accordance with one's type, such as when a person with a vegetarian-type metabolism eats a strict vegetarian diet. It can also be used as a balancing agent. If the autonomic nervous system is severely out of balance, diet can be used as a compensatory factor; a sympathetic-dominant person with an exhausted endocrine system might, for example, be advised to eat some meat in order to stimulate faster repair of those glands. This "balancing act," though, is a sophisticated, delicate procedure, and is recommended only under the care of a trained metabolic physician. Most patients are simply advised to eat the foods that are in natural accord with their own metabolisms.

Diet affects the autonomic nervous system biochemically, and in a number of other ways. One example of its effect on the nervous system is exhibited by the acid/alkaline balance. When the blood and cellular pH become more acid, or below approximately 7.4, the activity of the sympathetic nervous system is favored. A lower pH activates the influx of calcium and phosphorus into each cell, and increased calcium and phosphorus trigger release of the adrenergic nerve transmitters dopamine, epinephrine and norepinephrine, the major neurotransmitters of the sympathetic nervous system. Conversely, when the body becomes more alkaline, with a pH above 7.4, it favors the intracellular movement of potassium and magnesium, which potentiate acetylcholine, the major neurotransmitter of the parasympathetic nervous system.

Food supplements are a dietary means of improving balance of the autonomic nervous system. People with different metabolisms need different supplements. A sympathetic dominant person, for example, who already has relatively poor stimulation to the bowels and therefore is prone to constipation, is advised against taking iron supplements, which can accentuate constipation. Observations of people on nutritional programs indicate that in relation to the vitamin B and C complexes, sympathetic dominant people receive the greatest benefit from, among other supplements, ascorbic acid, thiamine, niacin, and pyridoxine, while parasympathetic types do best on sodium ascorbate, calcium ascorbate, pantothenic acid, inositol, choline and certain other vitamins and minerals. Sympathetic types, because of their decreased digestive activity, tend to need more digestive enzymes and hydrochloric acid.

One Man's Meat . . .

A number of varied diets are recommended to patients, based on each person's own individual needs. Along with a wide variety of diets, an endless combination of food supplements should be recommended.

Metabolic typing categorizes patients in numbers "1" through "10." Number "1" is the most extreme vegetarian type, the person who slowly burns even foods composed mostly of easily-digested carbohydrates, such as fruits, and rarely if ever craves or needs meat. The less extreme vegetarian types are "4s," who need some fish and fowl, and "6s," who metabolize food poorly and need to have more than half their food cooked, as well as much heavier support with supplements.

The most pronounced meat-eating types are "2s," who metabolize food so quickly that they need generous amounts of meat and other animal protein merely to avoid hypoglycemia. They seek out foods that will "stick to their ribs." The other carnivores, or parasympathetic dominant types, are "5s," who can eat a wide variety of foods, and "7s," who metabolize food poorly and often feel sluggish.

Balanced sympathetic/parasympathetic types are "3s," "8s," "9s" and "10s." At the bottom of the scale in terms of efficiency are the "3s," who have difficulty getting nutritional value out of their foods and require copious supplementation. At the top of the scale are the "10s." If there is a "perfect" metabolism, the "10s" have it. They can be healthy on a minimum of food and can glean abundant energy from every bite.

Changing Metabolic Types

Frequently, metabolic requirements change during the course of therapy, as a response to dietary change and the changing nature of the illness. An example of this occurred in the case of Mrs. G. G., 35, of Salt Lake City, who was diagnosed by her physician as having lung cancer in June of 1976. She was so short of breath she was confined to a wheelchair. She began radiation for the cancer, and was told that with chemotherapy she might live a year. Without chemotherapy, she was told, she would live about four months. She started a metabolic program in August 1976, and discontinued all other therapy. She had a sympathetic dominant metabolism, and needed only moderate amounts of meat, mostly fish or fowl, around mid-day. She had been eating a very poor diet, one too high in refined carbohydrates, which she, like most people, just couldn't metabolize. She began to feel better on this type of diet, but after several months she developed a severe cough, which sometimes happens when the parasympathetic branch begins to dominate. She was tested again after six months and was found to have shifted to parasympathetic dominance. Her diet was adjusted accordingly. When this was done, the cough and other symptoms she'd developed went away immediately. X-rays in May of 1977 showed she had no evidence of tumors. An individualized diet, suited to her metabolism, was, of course, only part of her recovery program. But, without it, it is doubtful that she would have been able to recover.

Individualizing the Entire Program

Dietary individualization, with simultaneous individualization of supplementation, is considered the most vital aspect of individualizing the whole program, but the other aspects are also important.

The other aspects of a complete program—detoxification, structural and emotional therapies and lifestyle change—are usually naturally tailored to individual needs.

Detoxification is the most uniform of all aspects of a complete metabolic program. Almost all people who are ill are advised to do coffee enemas, liver and gall bladder flushes, controlled sweating and dry skin brushing. Frequency is the major variable; a person with an advanced cancer, certain to be very toxic, may need to do as many as two or three coffee enemas daily. A person with only a moderately toxic condition would require a much less intensive detoxification program.

Structural and emotional therapies, of course, are almost always performed on an individualized basis. People are advised to find their own structural and emotional therapists, after a need for one has been determined. Many patients go to several different kinds of structural therapists, including chiropractors, osteopaths, masseusses, cranial specialists, reflexologists, spinal column stressologists and mandibular equilibration therapists. They also consult a variety of emotional therapists, including talk-oriented psychologists, bodywork-oriented psychologists, nutrition-oriented psychotherapists, primal-based therapists, relationship counselors, Freudian psychoanalysts, etc. People should find a professional that they feel comfortable with, can afford, and from whom they seem to derive benefit.

Lifestyle changes, too, should be highly individualized. Each person has his or her own peculiar mix of good and bad habits, and each person must apply himself or herself to the essentially self-sponsored discipline of changing habits.

If every segment of a person's program is highly individualized, he or she appears to stand an excellent chance of recovery. Each individualized segment of a metabolic program works synergistically with each other segment. Individualized diet works with individualized supplementation, both of which augment the benefits of an individualized emotional therapy program, and so on. Individualization makes every link in the chain of healing influences stronger.

Once this strong chain of healing influences has been established, even relentless diseases, such as cancer, can often be overcome.

CHAPTER ELEVEN

The Anti-Cancer Diet

"Historically," Dr. Peggy Fry of the University of Texas recently told a U.S. Senate Hearing, "the role of diet and nutrition in cancer therapy has been ignored."[1] This is an understatement. Nutritional therapy for cancer has not only been ignored, but actually villified by most cancer therapists, to the enormous detriment of their patients.

A vast body of research, however, supports the theory that a proper dietary component is the single most helpful part of a proper anti-cancer program. This theory has been put to the test by thousands of cancer patients who have used metabolic recovery programs, and evidence thus far gleaned from these thousands of cases indicates that the theory is correct.

Dr. Fry told the Senate that "If one believes the recent scientific literature, it is likely that nutritional support of cancer patients may provide more benefit than any other regime proposed in the last 30 years.[2] In spite of statements similar to this made by many other cancer researchers over the years, the National Cancer Institute still refuses to seriously study the power of nutritional therapy for malignancy. Only $10 million of the institute's $900 million budget is related to the study of nutrition, and virtually all of that is allocated to the division of Prevention and Causation, rather than the division of Cancer Treatment.

The N.C.I. has not always ignored the therapeutic powers of diet for cancer. According to one of the founders of the N.C.I., Dr. Dean Burk, "In the 1940s, one third to one half of N.C.I. sponsored research on cancer concerned diet. We 'breathed' diet then, even more than N.C.I. 'breathes' virus now." Dr. Burk told medical investigator Peter Barry Chowka that the N.C.I. largely dropped the study of nutritional therapy after World War II. "After World War II, along came chemotherapy, and in the early 1950s the virus program diverted attention away from diet."[3]

Former Senator Birch Bayh's wife, Marvella, representing the American Cancer Society, recently expressed to the U.S. Senate her dismay over the lack of knowledge most cancer therapists have about nutrition. "I'm told that few medical schools stress the importance of nutrition in training our doctors. Even my new car comes with a maintenance manual telling me what kind of fuel to feed it."[4] About a year later, Mrs. Bayh was dead, from cancer.

Diet and Cancer

A special anti-cancer diet, when properly individualized, performs two basic functions in opposing cancer. It provides a rapid influx of nutrients, and it helps to detoxify the body.

Metabolic doctors believe that an increased influx of nutrients can stimulate the immune system, can have a direct anti-tumoral effect, can improve the function of the entire system (boosting general resistance, balancing endocrine function, restoring weight loss, etc.), and can help prevent growth of new cancer cells. The detoxifying activities of diet include the neutralizing of toxins that contribute to further cancer cell growth (as well as the neutralizing of toxins that result from tumors), and the flushing away of toxins from the organs of elimination. All of these functions are highly important to a person who hangs in a precarious balance between life and death, and who is in particularly desperate need of stimulated immune and eliminative function.

The benefits of flooding the body with nutrition are almost impossible to exaggerate. University of Alabama research doctors Cheraskin, Ringsdorf and Clark, in *Diet and Disease,* cite no fewer than 85 laboratory animal experiments done within the last 25 years in which diet alone was employed to inhibit malignant growth.[5] These experiments were conducted on animals with cancers of the liver, gall bladder, skin, lung, kidney and breast. Among several dietary changes made were restricting calories, lowering protein and fat intake, improving the general quality of food, and providing food with enhanced vitamin and mineral content. They reported evidence of frequent "inhibitory effect on mitotic activity, including that of the latent cancer cell, and the limited ability of the tumor cells to compete with normal ones in the critical period. . . ."[6]

Some of the experiments cited by Cheraskin, Ringsdorf and Clark appear to indicate that many of the same activities of nutrients in preventing cancer can also help the body rid itself of cancer. Cheraskin, Ringsdorf and Clark cite thirteen recent experiments where nutritional therapy was successfully applied to cancer in humans. The cancers the people had included leukemia, alimentary tract cancer, neuroblastoma, choriocarcinoma, and breast cancer. These experiments included, among other things, use of restricted protein, high doses of vitamins and minerals, and general dietary improvement.

There have been other studies proving the value of nutritional therapy for cancer patients, including the very well-known studies by Drs. Linus Pauling and Ewan Cameron with vitamin C, which showed that use of large doses of the vitamin improved patient survival rates considerably, theoretically because the vitamin helped the immune system "recognize" the "foreign invader" and also helped neutralize the effects of toxic agents in patients' bodies. "The simplest and safest way to enhance immunocompetence in patients . . . is to increase their intake of vitamin C," wrote the doctors.[7]

Pauling and Cameron also show that improved nutrition can help the body resist the invasion of cancer cells by strengthening the resistance of normal cells. This is done by giving the normal cells nutrients that deactivate an enzyme in cancer cells, hyaluronidase, which cancer cells use to break down healthy cell walls prior to invasion.

Other enzymes found in foods, as was mentioned in earlier chapters, seem to have a direct anti-tumoral effect. These enzymes, including trypsin and chymotrypsin, are thought to help break down cancer cell walls, so that the immune system can penetrate and kill them. Other nutrients, including "anti-oxidants" such as vitamin E, act directly upon tumors by inhibiting their fermentation process, which is how many cancer cells "breathe."

The role in detoxification that diet can play is probably less important than the role played by flooding the body with nutrients, but it is still important.

Stimulating the kidneys with liquids and the intestine with additional dietary bulk, chiefly fiber, expedites removal of waste from the body. In a recovering cancer patient, whose body is constantly under the stress of toxicity from dead tumor cells, this is crucial. If these toxins remain for an extended time in the organs of elimination, they can re-enter the system, can cause a slowing down of the tumor-killing processes of the immune system, and can even create so serious a backlog of poisonous build-up that the patient can become overtly toxic and die.

Detoxification can also be aided at the intracellular level by diet. Certain nutrients can neutralize the toxins that have created the malignancy (and may be contributing to further cancer growth), as well as toxins that weaken all the systems of the body, and toxins that may come directly from the tumor itself.

Innumerable studies and experiments, as well as the clinical experiences of our colleagues in metabolic therapy, all support the thesis that proper diet can diminish existing malignancy.

Special Diets

Rule Number One given by metabolic doctors to cancer patients is: "Eat!" Too many cancer patients, failing to recognize the importance of nutrition (and receiving no encouragement to eat well from their physicians), simply refuse to eat enough. Cancer often causes a loss of appetite, possibly because of biochemical changes that relate to the taste buds, because of emotional upset, because of toxicity, because of liver dysfunction, and because of the appetite-killing treatments that often accompany the disease.

While many cancer patients are eating poorly, their tumors are "eating" well—their tumors are "devouring" the few nutrients that these patients metabolize.

A frequent result of inadequate nutrition is gradual starvation, or "cachexia," which kills about 30 per cent of all cancer patients,[8] more patients than any of the other most common direct causes of cancer death (which include infection, reaction to treatment, and organ failure due to impact of tumors, in that order).[9]

Dr. Peggy Fry says that "the do-nothing approach" of most institutions for the problem of cachexia "amounts to a defacto acceptance of patient starvation as ethical medical practice."[10] In an attempt at the Washington University School of Medicine to fight the problem of cachexia, 64 patients, bedridden and very near death, were put on continuous intravenous feeding with special vitamins, minerals and proteins. Almost all of them "were rehabilitated for a period of many months," and were "stronger," "happier" and "able to take care of themselves," according to Dr. Morton Pareira, who directed the experiment.[11]

Other patients, report Cheraskin, Ringsdorf and Clark, have shown slowing of tumor growth and stability of weight and strength while on a force-feeding program, but have rapidly deteriorated and shown acceleration of malignant growth when the program ended.[12]

The obvious moral of this for cancer patients is: "force-feed yourself." Most cancer patients would be wise to, as Hippocrates recommended, "let food be your medicine," and eat even if not particularly hungry.

Dietary Rules

People with cancer should not, though, eat whatever looks tasty. That habit contributes greatly to cancer causation, and, according to metabolic doctors, isn't going to contribute to a cancer remission.

People with cancer must show restraint and common sense. There are several terribly important rules for them to follow. These include: eat protein sparingly and on a time schedule; reduce consumption of fat, sugar and calories; eliminate intake of alcohol, highly processed and carcinogenic foods; and eat large amounts of foods high in easily-digested nutrients, such as fresh vegetables, fruits, grains and juices. Following these rules will, among other benefits, result in reduced stress on the liver, upon which the body's detoxification is dependent, and the pancreas, which must secrete the enzymes so vitally needed to break down cancer cell walls.

Sugar, fat, alcohol, excess calories and processed and carcinogenic foods will stress the liver, deterring it from its detoxification process. Sugar, as every diabetic knows, can greatly disturb the pancreas. Digestion of excessive protein can divert pancreatic enzymes from the tumor area, so proteins must be eaten sparingly, always with supplemental enzymes, and early in the day, so the body's enzymes will have a "rest" from digesting them. This interval of "rest" for the pancreas is very important. Too much consumption of fat can disturb hormonal levels, causing an excess secretion of estrogen, which appears to be implicated in causing many of the most common cancers.

High consumption of raw fruits and vegetables and their juices will afford the body a wealth of easily-digested vitamins, minerals and enzymes, as well as bulk and liquid to stimulate the eliminative organs. These foods will also biochemically shift the body to an alkaline condition, which tends to make the body's cells more permeable, allowing a more rapid influx of nutrients and egress of toxins. These foods will also, as described in the prior chapter, tend to shift the nervous system to a condition of parasympathetic dominance, which is a favorable condition for healing, since it creates increased nerve stimulation to some important organs and glands of the immune system, such as the thymus and liver.

A typical diet for a person with cancer, individualized according to that particular person's metabolic strengths and weaknesses, might include a daily fare of 70 per cent raw fruits and vegetables and fresh juices. This should be accompanied by whole grain products, dairy products (including cultured milk foods), up to two eggs a day, fish about twice a week (after four months), some seeds and nuts almost every day, and raw liver.

The food should be eaten in small quantities throughout the day, to ease digestion. Protein should be eaten in the morning, so that protein-digesting pancreatic enzymes will be freed in the afternoon and night for "digestion" of cancer cell walls. The foods should be eaten with digestive supplements and vitamins and minerals, which are, of course, a facet of diet, but will be discussed in a separate chapter for the sake of simplicity. Eating supplements with foods synergistically increases nutrient absorption. Food should be chewed very well, to aid digestion and stimulate enzyme production, and should not be eaten with liquids, which tend to dilute digestive secretions.

Organic, locally grown foods are far superior, since they will not have pollutants on or in them, which can greatly tax the liver, and because they are more likely to be grown in humus-rich, mineralized soil. Organic foods are less likely to be highly hybridized to increase size (at the expense of nutrient content), will almost certainly be fresher and will probably be field-ripened.

The benefits of foods without additives or pollutants appear to be authors to be considerable. The scientific community is generally divided on the question of possible harm from these toxic agents, because of uncertainty over the "dose-response" issue; they accept that these substances are poisons, they just don't know how much of the poison it takes to kill a person. With pesticides and herbicides on virtually every piece of produce in the supermarket, though, and with the average person now eating approximately five pounds of food additives per year, it seems probable to the authors that there is a sufficient "dose" of these pollutants to elicit a negative "response," particularly in a person teetering on the brink of death because of toxic overload and immune and eliminative weakness. If toxic chemicals used in farming were truly as benign as the agribusiness consortiums would like us to believe, then the farmers who use them probably wouldn't be dying at unprecedented rates of cancers of the "filtering" organs, including the kidneys and bladder, and from cancers of the blood (leukemia).

There has also been a powerful movement, financed and fueled by the gigantic food-processing industry, America's second-largest industry, to make Americans believe that the make-believe processed "food" jammed into metal cans and plastic containers is as nutritious as the real, unprocessed food coming straight from the earth. Real foods, regardless of what these people say, are better than pretend foods. Raw peas have three times the vitamin C and about twice the magnesium of canned peas, and one 1/100th the salt, to give just one very typical example. The potassium content of green beans plummets from 1,196 milligrams per 100 grams to 210 when they are canned, just as the vitamin C in them drops to one-tenth its uncanned amount. Many of the nutrient levels in whole wheat bread are 300 per cent higher than those found in white enriched bread. Canning commonly eradicates up to 80 per cent of the heat-destroyed vitamins, including some of the B vitamins, as well as many minerals.[13] Most processed foods, besides being de-natured and polluted, are filled with sugar; commercial catsups, to give one example, are commonly 33 per cent sugar. Other foods are loaded with lard and water to make them "filling."

Americans, who on the average eat 50 per cent of their food in its highly processed version,[14] have been literally "starving" for the past 40 years. It is our opinion, and that of many other researchers who have observed the degeneration of food and the inflation of degenerative disease rates since World War II, that a steep decline in our national health is the price we are collectively paying for eating "pretend" food instead of real food. The frightening increases in the incidence of childhood cancers and birth defects is but one index of this overall health decline.

Good, healthy diets do not require obsessive attention or ascetic denial. Diets recommended to cancer patients by metabolic physicians are probably the most strict and difficult of all health-stimulation diets to follow, but even these diets don't require much more than the elimination of protein intake. Even these relatively moderate diets become less stringent as the individual heals. It is, in fact, extremely important that additional protein be added as the person who is ill begins to heal, because protein depletions can be dangerous. The pancreas, for example, which the low-protein diet is designed to relieve, must have protein, as the cancer crisis abates, in order to rebuild its strength.

As a person overcomes cancer, his or her diet will tend to become increasingly more individualized. The initial dietary recommendations to people with cancer have many similarities, but these similarities begin to fade in the sixth to twelfth month of nutritional therapy. Natural carnivores, to give one obvious example, are advised to eat more meat than are natural vegetarians.

The diets for people with cancer, because they are intended to create a parasympathetic-dominant, alkaline condition to expedite healing, may cause patients to have some of the emotions generally associated with alkalinity, including depression and some degree of confusion. As long as the person with cancer recognizes this as a biochemically derived mental state, rather than a true mirror of one's outlook on life, the feelings can generally be tolerated. Often people with cancer begin their metabolic program with this kind of mental condition, because of neuro-toxicity and lack of nutrients reaching the brain, so they don't find it an additional burden. The feeling can usually be alleviated by temporarily reducing the amount of enzymes taken and by temporarily modifying the diet away from vegetarianism, which may be done as the program progresses.

The diet may also, if it is killing cancer cells, contribute to physical and mental feelings of toxicity by its destruction of tumor masses. If depression is a result of toxicity, it can usually be eliminated by a detoxifying procedure, such as a coffee enema.

There are no other significant side-effects from this nutritional program, unless one considers an occasional craving for chocolate cake a side-effect. In many cases, the diet begins to restore the patient's strength, feelings of well-being, and energy a few months after it is begun.

People who have had cancer are advised to remain on a healthy, whole foods diet for the rest of their lives. This healthy diet almost always becomes a desired habit for people who have had cancer, however, because of the pleasure derived from the vibrant, joyous feelings of health that the diet creates. People also commonly report that foods high in sugar, fat and processing do not taste very good after one gets out of the habit of eating them.

People with cancer have varying nutritional needs. These needs should be met with an individualized program devised by a physician who is competent in nutrition.

Following, however, are general guidelines applicable to many people who have cancer.

The Cancer Patient and Protein

Most foods, of course, contain protein, but in this section we will discuss high-protein foods.

High protein foods, eaten at breakfast and lunch only, may include dairy products, liver, and nuts and seeds. Protein, according to metabolic physicians who work with Dr. Kelley, should be restricted to about 30 grams daily in the first six months. More protein, including meats other than liver, may be added after about six months on the program. More protein may be eaten after six months of therapy because, by this time, pancreatic enzymes will not be needed quite so desperately to help break down cancer cells, and can be used to digest meat. Also, the pancreas, after six months of a low-protein diet, will begin to need some protein to rebuild itself.

Liver is acceptable because it is an excellent, highly nutritious blood-builder, and because of the theory, which metabolic doctors tend to believe is correct, that the substances composing the organs and glands of animals can, when eaten, stimulate and help to rebuild the corresponding organs and glands in humans.

When other meats are added to the diet, they also should be organic—raised without chemical growth-stimulants (particularly hormones) or antibiotics. The animals should have been raised on grass and untreated grain and allowed to graze and roam. Fish that are eaten should also be organically raised. Some commercially raised fish are fed pollutants, and some ocean fish come from polluted waters. Ascertaining purity of fish can be difficult, but knowledgeable proprietors of seafood shops can alert customers to locally grown, pure, fresh products.

Meat, say metabolic doctors, may be added to the diet when the person with cancer begins to exhibit a resistance to the disease. Fowl and extra fish should be added before beef, which is the hardest meat to digest. Low-fat meats should be sought; the average American eats 44 per cent of his or her diet as fat—a grossly excessive amount.[15] Organ meats are almost always preferable to muscular tissue meats, although they are higher in cholesterol and should be accompanied with lecithin supplements. It should be remembered that overcooking kills enzymes and other nutrients. Meat should always be accompanied with pancreatic enzymes and hydrochloric acid supplements, and often lecithin, and should be eaten before noon as long as there is any trace of malignancy, in order to give the pancreas and other organs an afternoon and evening "rest." One's metabolic type will determine relative need for meat as recovery occurs.

Some people become attached to vegetarianism for various reasons, some of which are irrational and emotional. Vegetarianism should be engaged in as a form of simple dietary manipulation, and not as a "religion" that one becomes compulsive about. Most Americans and Europeans have a genetic background peopled by carnivores, and this genetic heritage should not be ignored. Excessive meat-eating, the cause of so many of our degenerative disease problems, should not be countered with excessive meat avoidance.

Dairy products are a high-quality source of protein, almost as good as meat and somewhat easier to digest. Milk products, including raw cow's and goat's milk, buttermilk, yogurt, kefir, cottage cheese, brick cheese and Piima yogurt, may be combined to total eight ounces per day. Butter and cream, in strict moderation, may be used in addition to this. Two fertile eggs a day may be eaten, except by melanoma or leukemia patients.

Pasteurized milk, with some of its enzymes and nutrients removed by the process, should be replaced by raw milk. Goat's milk is often preferable to higher-fat cow's milk, one glass of which contains nine grams of fat and 160 calories.[16] The high female hormone, protein and fat content of milk products dictates against heavy consumption of them, especially during the early stages of therapy.

Yogurt, Piima yogurt (an easily-clabbering form of the product), and kefir (a cultured milk drink), are more easily digested than other dairy products because they are naturally fermented. The good cultured milk products contain lactobacillus acidophilus, a helpful bacteria that aids digestion of foods and synthesizes some important fractions of the B-complex. Some types of yogurt, developed at temperatures of 105 to 120 degrees Fahrenheit, have organisms that digest most other bacteria, both destructive and favorable. Kefir, made from fresh whole milk and kefir grains, has many of the same benefits for digestion. Buttermilk, too, can benefit the intestinal flora. Careful attention, though, should be paid to the quality of the product. Some commercial yogurts are nothing more than sugar-filled puddings which do more harm than good. There are several reputable brands, though, including "Continental." Yogurt and kefir can easily be made at home (see chapter addendum).

After six months on the nutritional therapy program, doctors allow cheese to be eaten in moderation before 3:00 p.m., since it is an excellent source of protein, natural fats, oils and minerals. Carnivorous metabolic types, such as "2s" and "5s," will enjoy this extra protein very much.

Some of the processed cheeses and some of the make-believe "cheese-like products" are just junk foods, but the raw milk, unpasteurized, undyed, fresh cheeses in health food, specialty and gourmet stores are superb foods. Excellent cheeses are made from raw milk during the young-grass months of Wisconsin, and from raw milk from cattle and goats fed on mineral-rich pastures where no chemical fertilizers, herbicides or pesticides are used. Cottage cheeses can be very beneficial, especially those made from raw unpasteurized milk, with lactobacillus acidophilus. Be careful in the reading of cheese labels. Many that claim to be "all natural" are highly processed foods.

It is extremely important for the person engaged in a serious nutritional therapy program to remember that junk food is found not only in fast-food restaurants, but also in fancy restaurants, delicatessens, on many supermarket shelves, and on the shelves of many so-called health food stores. Even mom's apple pie, as prepared by most mothers—with vats of fat and sugar—is junk food.

Raw nuts and seeds, including almonds, cashews, pecans, filberts, Brazil nuts, walnuts, sunflower seeds, pumpkin seeds and sesame seeds, may be eaten frequently, before 3:00 p.m., even during the first six months of the program, when protein is most highly restricted. They should be kept in a cool place, preferably the refrigerator. Some researchers don't recommend raw seeds or nuts, claiming that the enzyme inhibitors in them make digestion difficult. Others feel, though, that thorough mastication or overnight soaking nullifies the enzyme inhibitors.

A high-protein product that should be used sparingly is soy. Soy products tend to upset the acid/alkaline balance, they appear to inhibit enzyme systems, and they pose a threat of supplying the body with excess copper. Liquid lecithin derived from soybeans is a good product, though, and should be used frequently.

Eggs are a balanced protein, with all the essential amino acids in proper proportion. Two of them, according to metabolic doctors, can be eaten at any time during the day, by non-melanoma or leukemia patients. They should be fertilized, and should come from chickens that were allowd to live outdoors. If only unfertilized eggs from an agribusiness "egg-factory" are available, it is preferable to do without them. Eggs, though high in cholesterol, contain sufficient natural lecithin to counter-balance the cholesterol.

Thirty grams a day of protein, the recommended limit for cancer patients during their first six months on the program, is only about one-third the amount eaten by the average person in America.[17] During the second six months, protein intake may increase to a maximum of 45 grams per day, if the cancer is still a severe problem. If the severity of the disease appears to have waned, a minimum of 45 and a maximum of 60 grams is recommended. Parasympathetic, carnivore types are especially likely to need more complex protein after six months. A list of the various amounts of protein in foods can be found in many diet books.

This restricted amount of protein may be somewhat difficult for one to become adjusted to, but adherence to this rule is absolutely vital in order to achieve success.

The Cancer Patient and Carbohydrates

Extremely important for the recovering cancer patient is consumption of large quantities of unrefined, complex carbohydrates, such as those found in fresh fruits and vegetables and whole grains. Refined, simple carbohydrates, or sugar products, are, on the other hand, anathema to cancer patients. The poorly metabolizing metabolic types, the "3s," "6s," and "7s," have an incredibly difficult time digesting sugary, plastic, fabricated foods.

Unfortunately, most Americans eat far more refined carbohydrates and far fewer complex carbohydrates than they should. The Senate Subcommittee on Nutrition and Human Needs found in 1978 that consumption of complex carbohydrates had fallen from composing 37 per cent of total caloric intake in 1910 to only 21 per cent in 1976. Concurrently, consumption of simple carbohydrates had risen from 12 per cent to 18 per cent. When this is added to our average fat consumption, we see that the average American is living on a diet of 56 per cent straight fat and sugar.[18] For the cancer patient, this type of diet can be fatal. Sugar, which is very debilitating to the pancreas and stressful to the liver, should be carefully avoided.

Fresh fruits, vegetables and grains should compose most of the diet of a person with cancer. About 70 per cent of this food should be eaten raw, during the first six months of the program, by most patients. The raw vegetarian diet will provide a maximum of nutrients, especially enzymes, will help the organs of elimination, will be easily digested, and will shift the body into an alkaline, parasympathetic-dominant condition, which is favorable for healing. As the person who is ill recovers, the diet can be gradually shifted away from raw vegetarianism, but, for at least the first year, this type of diet should still predominate.

Vegetables may be eaten as salads, or can be steamed lightly, or cooked in some other way. Large bowls of salad should comprise the majority of all vegetables eaten, for reasons of nutrition, ease of digestion and elimination. A variety of salads, often ones made of fresh, raw vegetables that are not commonly thought of as salad vegetables, such as broccoli or cauliflower or asparagus, can keep this part of the regime from being boring. Innovative use of dressings, including the very healthful yogurt and oil and vinegar dressings, can relieve the monotony of frequent salads. Large salads often compose the main course of the cancer patient's evening meal, and can be made more interesting with side dishes of lightly steamed vegetables or grains or hot, toasted breads or rolls with butter or dressing. Seeds and nuts can also make salads more appealing. For salad ideas, write for *Diet and Salad Suggestions,* Dr. N. W. Walker, Norwalk Press, O'Sullivan and Woodside Co., 2218 E. Magnolia, Phoenix, AZ 85024. People with highly vegetarian-oriented metabolisms, though, will need almost no encouragement to eat their salads—these people are inveterate "rabbit food" eaters.

Care should be taken to avoid cottonseed oil dressings, because cotton is commonly sprayed with a variety of toxic chemicals. Better oils for dressing include unrefined sesame, olive, safflower, sunflower, walnut, apricot and almond oil, in that order. There are now several pure "prepared" salad dressings in health food stores, some of them dry-packaged so that a person's favorite oil can be added. Most commercial dressings, however, are just nicely packaged junk foods, including most of the "all natural" ones, which contain "all natural" white sugar.

Vegetables should be lightly steamed if cooked, or at least cooked in their own juices, which should also be eaten. Many enzymes are destroyed at 104 °F. and almost all are killed at 140 °F. One of the primary reasons for the inclusion of cooked foods in the anti-cancer diet is simply because most people are unwilling to eat a totally raw diet. Some foods, though, such as rice or other grains, can be difficult to eat raw, and a few foods actually yield more vitamins when cooked. Carrots, for example, have a higher vitamin C yield when cooked because certain tissues are broken down.

Vegetables provide a bounty of nutrients. Vegetables exceptionally high in vitamins C and A, which are immune-supportive and natural detoxifiers, include artichokes, asparagus, green beans, beets, broccoli, cabbage, carrots, cauliflower, chard, chicory, corn, kale, romaine lettuce, onions, peas, peppers, potatoes, spinach, sweet potatoes and tomatoes.[19] Actually, virtually all fresh, whole vegetables are rich sources of nutrients, and can be used in wide, changing varieties.

Fruits are equally as easy to digest, and provide immense amounts of vitamins, minerals and enzymes, particularly A, C, potassium, calcium and phosphorus.[20] People with cancer may eat as many raw fruits as desired, not only for their nutrient value, but also because they have the reputation for being the most internally cleansing of all foods (because of their high fiber, liquid and enzyme content). They should be eaten raw, as ripe as possible, and should be kept at room temperature. Bananas, to maximize ripeness, which potentiates nutrient values, should not be eaten until the green has disappeared from the tips and several brown spots appear on the peels.

Fruits are also excellent at alkalinizing the body's pH, thereby helping shift it into a parasympathetic-dominant condition. All natural acids exert an alkalinizing effect on the body, and the natural acids found in fruits include citric, malic, tartaric and oxalic acids.

These acids are also, according to writer and teacher Jethro

Kloss, germicidal, antibacterial and antiviral. Kloss maintains that "A fruit diet will disinfect the stomach and alimentary canal."[21] Also, Kloss says, oxalic acid, found in plums, tomatoes and rhubarb, is a stimulant to both the colon and the liver.[22]

Most of the common fruits contain these acids; fruits especially high in them are apples, apricots, pears, peaches, cherries, grapefruit, grapes, strawberries, raspberries, lemons, limes, oranges, currants, blackberries and gooseberries.[23]

Fruits containing high amounts of vitamins A and C, which are particularly helpful for the cancer patient, include apples, apricots, bananas, blackberries, grapefruit, lemons, limes, mangoes, melons, nectarines, oranges, papayas, peaches, tangerines and strawberries.[24]

Papayas are a superb source of digestive enzymes. Most digestive enzymes found in health food stores, as well as meat tenderizers found in grocery stores, contain high amounts of papaya. A moderate amount of ripe papaya every day can be very helpful to the cancer patient, according to metabolic physicians..

Dried fruits are more nutrient-filled than canned or frozen fruits, and can make very good snacks when mixed with nuts. If possible, organic fruits should be eaten. If vegetables and fruits are not organic, soak them overnight before eating (see addendum).

Metabolic doctors say that juices of organic fruits and vegetables are absolutely essential to an anti-cancer diet. They are unmatched in providing concentrated nutrients, including unharmed enzymes, and in helping provide detoxification to the liver, kidneys and colon. Cancer immunotherapist Virginia Livingston, M.D., says, "The very ill need vegetable juices primarily." She counsels patients to "drink juices as often as you can, as much as one quart of carrot juice each day."[25] She recommends most highly juices of the apple, carrot, cabbage, tomato, cucumber, spinach and beet. She recommends mixing equal parts carrot and apple juice; and three parts carrot to one part spinach; and three parts carrot to one part cabbage; and equal parts tomato and carrot; and four parts carrot, two parts cucumber and one part beet.[26] Doctors have found carrot juice, with its high vitamin A content, to be excellent for all cancer patients, who are also advised to drink several glasses of green juice daily for its alkalinizing effect and nutrients. Hypoglycemic patients, though, are advised to restrict use of sweet and green juices.

Patients on Hippocrates Health Institute anti-cancer diets are advised to drink several glasses of wheat grass juice daily. This juice is an excellent alkalinizer and detoxifier and is full of vitamins and minerals. Patients on Gerson anti-cancer programs are advised to drink ten eight-ounce glasses daily of orange, apple, carrot and green-vegetable juices, or about one glass every hour throughout the day. Dr. Gerson's diet commonly calls for use of as much as 1800 pounds of carrots and 1300 pounds of apples per year, mostly for juice.[27] Most practitioners who recommend juice insist that patients use fresh, organic fruits and vegetables. Use of a high-quality juicer, such as the "Acme" or "Champion" brands, maximizes nutrients gleaned and minimizes enzymes destroyed.

Juices have a very valuable function, but metabolic doctors feel that one must not rely upon them, as some nutrition-based cancer therapies do, too heavily. The cancer patient, especially once his or her healing is well established, needs a higher-protein, more acidic diet than that which is afforded by extreme reliance upon juice, or even juice with fruits and vegetables. The superbly metabolizing type "10" can live indefinitely on this sort of vegetarian/fruitarian diet, but these extremely healthy people rarely seem to contract cancer.

Whole grains provide an important source of protein to the cancer patient's meat-restricted diet. Wheat, millet, barley, buckwheat, oats, rice, rye and corn are rich in nutrients and fiber. Using the entire grain is of the utmost importance, since nearly all of the B and E vitamins, unsaturated fatty acids, and many of the amino acids are removed in the refining process.[28] Grains that are stripped of nutrients and then artificially "enriched" are enriched with only about one-sixth of the B-vitamins, most of the iron, and none of the other minerals or proteins that were removed.[29] Refined grains are inordinately harder to digest and metabolize, because of their "gluey" texture, and they block the absorption of other nutrients by forming a coating on the wall of the intestine. Most white flours are merely wheat endosperm, with all the bran and germ removed, lacking as much as 80 per cent of the original nutrients.[30] Bran is also well-known as the highest of high fiber foods, which "scour" the intestinal walls of the coating that blocks nutrient absorption.

Whole grains are especially rich in vitamins B and E, calcium, lecithin, zinc, copper and iodine. The bioflavonoid "rutin," found in high quantities in several grains, is very helpful in speeding the clotting of internal hemorrhage. Some grains, including millet, are intestinal lubricants, which aid bowel transit time and help natural detoxification.[31]

People with cancer are advised to have a raw, whole-grain cereal almost every morning. It should include equal parts wheat berries, buckwheat, rye, barley, oat groats, millet, sesame seeds, brown rice, flaxseed, corn, alfalfa seeds, lentils, mung beans and almonds (see chapter addendum).

People are advised to sprout seeds and grains, or buy sprouts if fresh, organic ones can be found. A seed is at its peak of vitality, in terms of nutrient content, during the sprouting phase. People with cancer are allowed to eat no more than one cup of sprouts per day, because sprouts, especially if too mature, can exert an antienzyme effect. Sprouts may be eaten at any time during the day, and are often good mixed into salads (see addendum).

The fruits, vegetables and juices that compose the basis of this diet are said to seem after a short time to be fulfilling, deliciously variant in taste and texture, and richly provident in energy. People with sympathetic-dominant, natural vegetarian metabolisms tend to become extremely fond of this type of diet, and are advised to continue it indefinitely.

Fats and Oils

When used in moderation and in their natural form, fats and oils are a valuable addition to the diet, even a low-fat, anti-cancer diet. Unsaturated fatty acids play an important role in thyroid function by combining with iodine to release it slowly. "Fats," wrote nutritional writer Adelle Davis, "are needed to . . . stimulate bile flow."[32] Fats and oils supply many nutrients, including vitamins D, F, E and linoleic acid, and provide energy stability because they are so slowly oxidized. Fats help make calcium available to cells and seem to help protect against radiation.[33]

Fats, of course, are one of our overweight society's favorite "whipping boys," blamed for much of our cancer and cardiovascular disease. Overconsumption of them is the real culprit, though. There is also a generally poor appreciation of quality differences in fats and oils.

People are told by metabolic doctors to avoid margarines and most vegetable oils, because they are hydrogenated and made into artificially saturated fats. All margarines are also injected with yellow dye.

The best fats and oils come in nuts and seeds, which contain all the naturally occurring vitamins, minerals, enzymes and proteins needed to digest, metabolize and excrete the fats and oils. Sprouted, soaked or freshly ground grains are very good sources of oils.

Small quantities of liquid oils, unrefined, cold-pressed and refrigerated, add variety and goodness to the other foods recommended. Any natural fat, whether from meat, poultry or vegetables, will be a soft golden color and will melt at room temperature. All natural fats and oils become rancid easily.

Desirable natural fats and oils include cod and halibut oil, coconut oil when it comes from freshly grated coconut, flaxseed, safflower and sunflower oils, and raw, undyed butter and cream. If these products are used with restraint, they will improve an anti-cancer diet immeasurably. They will be of special value to parasympathetic carnivores, particularly as their malignancies recede, because these people need the slow-oxidizing qualities of fats and oils.

Forbidden Foods

Other than sugar, highly refined foods and polluted foods, the only other common dietary components that people with cancer should avoid are caffeinated and alcoholic beverages, and chlorinated and fluoridated water.

Alcohol is said to be entirely incompatible with an anti-cancer program. One drink, of course, will not derail an entire metabolic program, but alcohol, for a person with cancer, is believed to be one of the worst single substances that could be ingested. Alcohol's major negative impact is upon the liver, which is of vital importance to the recovering cancer patient. Alcohol stresses the liver more than any other food or drink that may be taken into the body, with the possible exception of extremely polluted foods, some pharmaceutical drugs (including some chemotherapy agents), and some illegal drugs. Alcohol restricts the blood flow in the capillaries, toxifies the entire system, leeches nutrients from the bloodstream and cells, is extremely hard to digest, can deprive the brain of oxygen, depresses the central and autonomic nervous systems, and frequently depresses the emotions. Alcohol consumption was proven by Dr. Roger Williams to increase deaths not just from cancers of the esophagus, to which consumption has been directly linked, but also cancers of the breast, thyroid and skin. This apparently occurs because of the harm alcohol causes the entire system.

Cancer patients who are drinkers are advised to stop drinking completely during at least their first six months on the program, and to indulge in alcohol in strict moderation only after their cancer crisis is well past.

Caffeinated drinks are considered less harmful, but still wreak havoc upon the nervous system, pancreas, adrenal glands, thyroid, stomach and emotions. Caffeine can make the body temporarily flooded with sucrose, by stimulating the pancreas, and can shift the body to a sympathetic-dominant, acidic condition. Both these conditions may be temporarily pleasant. The pendulum of biochemical balance is predetermined to swing back, however, leaving the patient hungry, tired, nervous, and weakened in several vital organs and glands. Almost all non-organic coffee, also, is sprayed with insecticides, and can be highly toxic.[34]

People with cancer are told by metabolic doctors to substitute herbal and other drinks for coffee, tea and caffeinated soft drinks during their recuperative phase, and to thereafter use these beverages in very limited quantities.

Fluoride, added to drinking water, has been proven toxic by, among others, National Cancer Institute co-founder Dr. Dean Burk and Dr. John Yiamouyiannis. Virtually every clinical ecologist in America agrees that fluoride, even at the supposedly safe dose of one part per million parts of water, is directly irritating and carcinogenic to the lining of the gastrointestinal tract, and toxic to the entire system.[35] Drs. Burk and Yiamouyiannis, citing epidemiological studies, showed that consumption of fluoridated water increases cancer death by an average of 23 per cent.[36] Drs. I. H. Herskowitz and I. C. Norton of St. Louis University reported in the 1960s that fluoride ingestion in fruit flies increased tumor incidence from 12 to 100 per cent.[37] N. C. Taylor at the University of Texas showed that one part per million fluoride increased cancer deaths in white mice by 17 per cent.[38]

Chlorine added to water has similarly been demonstrated to be a factor in increased cancer deaths. A recent U.S. government study of cities with chlorinated water supplies showed that these cities invariably had higher cancer rates than non-chlorinated cities. Chlorination has been shown in experiments to destroy vitamin E.

Other pollutants are commonly found in the drinking water of cities, including germs, acids, human excrement and industrial wastes.

People with cancer are advised to buy a good water distiller to clean their tap water, or should drink distilled water. It is important to use a good distiller, such as a "New World," rather than to use an ineffective charcoal-filter that attaches to the faucet and only removes solid particles.

All patients, regardless of metabolic type, are advised to avoid these harmful substances.

A Small Sacrifice

As we've shown, an anti-cancer diet is neither highly restrictive nor devoid of foods that please the palate.

Eydie Mae, in *How I Conquered Cancer Naturally,* describes her reaction to going on a health-promoting diet. "One of the things we learned was that our 'living foods' diet was not as revolutionary as we had originally thought. . . . No matter where we went, our request for a fresh fruit meal or a raw vegetable meal was met with very little surprise. It just wasn't difficult.

"We have come to thoroughly enjoy eating this way. I found that I wasn't going to give up anything of importance."[39]

Most patients, once their health returns, no longer need an

individualized anti-cancer diet to counter malignancy, but eat one nonetheless. To them, the thought of returning to a diet dictated by Betty Crocker and Colonel Sanders is repugnant. People with cancer soon find, after beginning this diet, that, after eating real food, pretend food never tastes the same again.

(Chapter Addendum)

Extra Information On Diet

"Special Preparation of Foods"

Preparing Kefir

Kefir is a cultured milk beverage made with fresh whole milk and kefir grains. These grains are small colonies of milk-fermenting yeasts and bacteria. They resemble cooked rice clumps. Once the grains are obtained, the culture can be kept growing for years.

The grains may be dried and stored. It is wise to have a few tucked away for emergency use or for providing someone else with a starter. Some health food stores stock them.

To make the beverage, put 4 or more ounces of kefir grains in 1 quart of whole raw milk. This mixture should stand at room temperature for at least twelve hours. If a more tart beverage is desired, it can stand for a longer time. The grains should be strained out and the beverage chilled. The grains are now ready to be added to a fresh jar of milk. To keep grains, place them in fresh milk and set them in the refrigerator until needed.

Preparing Cottage Cheese

Two quarts of raw milk should sit at room temperature until clabbered, or "set." The clabbered milk should be heated very slowly, in a pan with water, on the lowest setting, until whey begins to come to the top. It should be allowed to sit for ten minutes, then drained through a fine sieve—or through two thicknesses of nylon net lining a colander, or fastened to a small pail with several clean clothespins. The cheese should be seasoned with a high-quality salt product, such as Ultra-Salt, and have a little cream added at serving time. To speed the process, add 2 to 3 tablespoons of buttermilk or yogurt to the milk and allow the mixture to remain at room temperature until set. Then proceed with the prior directions.

Preparing Butter and Buttermilk

Use raw goat's or cow's milk if possible. Leave it in the refrigerator for approximately a day, or until the cream rises to the top. The cream should then be skimmed off and allowed to age another day in the refrigerator. Pour cream into a blender until it is a little over half full. Turning the blender on and off, blend the cream until it gets thicker and forms small grains (rich cream immediately forms butter). The volume will increase until it almost fills the blender, and then little grains of butter will begin to separate from the buttermilk. Stop the blender and use a rubber scraper to help form the butter into lumps that can be removed. Place the butter in a bowl that has been scalded and rinsed with cold water. The buttermilk should be poured off through a small strainer, if one wishes to remove every bit of butter. Some people prefer buttermilk with a few golden specks of butter left in. The buttermilk should be chilled to drink. Use the rubber scraper to "work" the butter, smoothing, turning, and pressing it to take out remaining buttermilk. The butter should be rinsed in cold water and worked again until the water runs clear. One-fourth teaspoon of a high quality salt product should be added for every half pound of butter, and mixed well.

Buttermilk—suggestions for use:

1. May be mixed with tomato juice, half and half, for a refreshingly different drink.

2. May be blended with any fruit or fruit juice, adding brewer's yeast, lecithin, or kelp for added nutrients—a delicious snack-time food.

3. May be used as all or part of the liquid in Knox or Grayslake gelatin desserts—especially good with berries or peaches.

4. May be served with baked potato as a tangy topping.

5. May be used as a delicious ingredient in salad dressings, adding herbs, tomatoes, onions and oil to suit one's taste.

6. Excellent just as it is for a drink or between-meal snack food.

Preparing Non-Organic Vegetables and Fruits

If it is necessary to use fresh vegetables and fruits that have been sprayed with herbicides or pesticides, we recommend soaking them in one-fourth cup of apple cider vinegar per sink full of water before refrigerating, for 30 minutes. There are other food cleansers on the market that are supposed to be organic, but we suggest checking the ingredients carefully before buying. If ingredients are not fully listed, or if one is in doubt after reading the list, the vinegar should be used.

Preparing Eggs

The egg must be heated in the shell at a temperature of 140 °F. to 160 °F. (the normal temperature of very hot tap water) for five minutes before it is cracked. This destroys an enzyme just inside the membrane, under the shell, that prevents the biotin in the egg from functioning normally. When biotin functions properly, it greatly reduces the cholesterol risks of eggs.

After the preheating of the eggs, before cracking them, they may be fixed and eaten in any way desired. Soft-boiled and raw eggs are preferable, though it isn't absolutely necessary to eat them in these forms. For those eating as much raw food as possible, we suggest eating the eggs raw in a blended drink of some kind, flavored to suit one's taste.

Preparing Beans

Dry beans of all types are good sources of food for the cancer patient, and may be used two or three times a week at any time of the day. One of the best ways we have found to prepare them is to cook them at a temperature of 250 °F. We place 2 cups of dried, washed beans in a bean pot—to which we add 5 cups of distilled water, 5 garlic cloves, 2 tablespoons of olive oil, 1 teaspoon of a high-quality salt product such as Ultra-Salt, or kelp, and one-eighth teaspoon of cayenne pepper, plus any other desired seasoning. Place the pot, covered, in an oven overnight at 250 °F.

There are many other good, healthful ways of preparing beans as a tasty addition to the diet.

Preparing Piima Yogurt

Yogurt is a protein source, and a source of helpful bacteria that can synthesize some important fractions of the B complex. Such bacteria cannot grow without some fat, so this is one good reason for using whole milk rather than skim in the yogurt. Milk sugar is used up in the development of the bacteria, making the yogurt attractive to weight watchers.

Cultured products tend to be compatible with other necessary organisms in the body. They are thus of great value in human nutrition and should be used generously and often. It has been found that certain heat-cultured yogurts, developed at temperatures of 105° to 120 °F., have organisms that digest most other intestinal bacteria—both destructive and favorable. Instead of these, use Continental Yogurt, if a commercial source is used, and room-temperature (70° to 90 °F.) cultures, such as Piima, if homemade products are used. One can obtain Continental Yogurt from the health food store, and can use that as the starter in homemade yogurt.

A heaping tablespoon of Piima starter (available, freeze-dried, at Piima, Box 2614, La Mesa, CA 92041, $3.00), should be put into a wide-mouth jar, with a cup of whole raw milk, at room temperature. The mixture should be stirred until it is smooth and thin. Raw cow's milk is preferable; because raw goat's milk may not thicken properly, depending on what the goat has eaten. Pasteurized, canned, or powdered milk can be used, but fresh milk is preferable. Milk is best at room temperature but will also work if cold. It should not be heated.

After one-half hour, the jar should be covered, with light excluded, and placed in an approximately 70° temperature. After eight hours, the mixture should be checked to see if it has reached proper consistency. If not, it should be cultured until it does, but not over 24 hours. If the mixture is shaken or stirred, it will separate into curds and whey. The more quickly it cultures, the sweeter it will be. When the Piima has reached the right custard-like consistency, it is ready.

Each individual jar of yogurt should contain the amount that is likely to be consumed in a one-day period (half pint, pint, or quart). If not to be used at once, the yogurt should be refrigerated. It will keep this way for a week or more. Each batch should include an extra jar to use as the starter for the next batch. This, too, should be refrigerated if not immediately used. The starter should always be taken from a fresh jar, rather than from the remainder in a bottle that has been used, which may have become contaminated by the spoons dipped into it or by airborne bacteria.

Piima is delicious as is, or served as a sundae with fresh fruit or natural fruit concentrates. Piima makes an excellent sour cream, if heavy cream, rather than milk, is used in a recipe. Cream cheese can be made from the cream Piima, depending on the thickness of the cream and the length of culturing time. Baked potatoes can be served with either milk or cream Piima.

Preparing Sprouts

Select quality seeds for sprouting—ones that have not been treated with chemicals. The sprouts will be no better than the seeds one starts with. It is not recommended that chloride of lime be used on them, which is often suggested as a mold inhibitor.

There are various good sprouting devices available at health food stores. One of the easiest methods for successful sprouting is simply to use a one-quart glass jar with a wide mouth, a small piece of nylon net (stocking remnants are excellent) or a stainless steel strainer top that screws onto the jar (available at some health food stores), and a rubber band (if one uses the nylon net).

Alfalfa seeds and mung beans are the easiest to sprout, so a beginner might start with either of these. In one or two trials one usually masters the technique. Place 1 rounded tablespoon of alfalfa seeds in a one-quart, wide-mouth glass jar, with 2 to 3 inches of distilled water covering the seeds. One-half teaspoon of granulated, dried kelp may be added to the water to increase the minerals in the sprouts, and the seeds should be soaked in this solution one day or overnight. Cover the jar with nylon net or strainer-top during this soaking period, leaving off the solid lid to use for storing sprouts in the refrigerator.

After the seeds have soaked, pour off any excess water through the strainer top or nylon net. (Soaking and rinse waters should be saved, since they are extremely rich in minerals and other valuable nutrients. They can be used in soups and beverages.) The seeds should be rinsed thoroughly in lukewarm water and drained well. They are now ready for sprouting.

Lay the jar on its side, at an angle, to insure further drainage through the netting or strainer top. Rinse the seeds twice daily by pouring lukewarm water through the netting or strainer top, swirling it around, and pouring the excess off. (Water for this purpose may be taken from the tap, though distilled water is preferred. Artificially softened water should not be used.) The seeds should be kept moist but not wet. They should be drained carefully after each rinsing, and the jar laid once again on its side at an angle. It is wise to keep the seeds at 72 °F., but if they are kept at a higher temperature, and if the air is dry, they may need a few extra rinses each day. The strainer top or net is left on throughout the sprouting process, providing plenty of ventilation.

After the seeds begin to sprout, they will discard their hulls. During rinsing, hulls have a tendency to float to the top. They can be removed with a colander as soon as the sprouts are large enough not to pass through the holes. Transfer the sprouts from the jar into the colander, and lift them carefully while pouring or running lukewarm water through them. Hulls will go through the holes in the colander and crisped sprouts will remain. Discard the loose hulls. When the jar is filled with water during rinsing, one can sometimes remove the net or strainer top and scoop the larger bean and seed hulls off the water surface with a spoon.

The sprouts should be rinsed morning and evening for about five days—at which time, depending on weather and temperature, tiny green leaves will crop up. Many people consider alfalfa sprouts "full grown" when the two small leaves are just starting to appear. But if growth goes on to the point where these first leaves are well formed, one may develop the chlorophyll in the sprouts. This is done by placing them, in their jar, near a window, in indirect sunlight for a day or more.

When one is ready to "harvest" the sprouts, they should be placed in a bowl of water, separated, and dropped back lightly into the jar a few at a time so they do not pack. The top should be replaced, all excess water drained off, and the jar laid on its side as before. In eight to twelve hours, one will find that the sprouts have filled the jar entirely. They are now ready to be eaten and can be stored in the refrigerator with closed jar lid for about a week. Another batch should be started right away, or a day before these are to be eaten.

Sometimes when one tries to sprout seeds, they do not germinate, or they begin to ferment, rot or mold. The trouble is usually due to one of these causes:

1. Seeds are old or have been improperly stored.
2. Too much water was used.
3. Insufficient water was used.
4. Temperature was too cold.
5. Too much light was allowed.
6. Not enough air was allowed in.

Preparing Whole Grain Cereal

The following grains, seeds, and nuts should be mixed together well in a large container (1 pound of each): wheat berries, buckwheat, rye, barley, oat groats, millet, sesame seeds, brown rice, flaxseed, corn, alfalfa seeds, lentils, mung beans and almonds. Store this mixture in the refrigerator. Each night, 3 or 4 tablespoons of the grains, seeds and nuts should be ground well in a seed mill, then barely covered with cream, or water, and pineapple or other fruit juice or natural flavoring. This should be allowed to stand at room temperature overnight. In the morning, fruit and/or honey, cream, black cherry concentrate, or any fruit juice or natural flavoring can be added to make the mixture delicious. This should be eaten raw.

Many people have problems waking up at night and not being able to go back to sleep, because they don't have enough "fuel," or blood sugar and protein, to carry them through the night. If this is the situation, one may eat the whole-grain cereal before bed, instead of at breakfast, to provide enough slow-burning carbohydrates and protein to carry one through the night.

If one does not find the mixture pleasing to the taste, one may start with four grains and add the others, one by one, as desired. One will be getting the optimum in nutritional contents, however, only if all fourteen grains are eaten.

(Chapter Addendum)

Extra Information On Diet

"Sample Menus For Two Days"

FIRST DAY

Upon Arising:
- 2 teaspoons Hawthorne berry tea
- Green vegetable juice

BREAKFAST
- Grain pancakes with raw butter and honey
- Fruit and pit jam
- Herb tea
- Carrot juice

SNACK
- Large glass of fruit juice

LUNCH
- Sauteed fish
- Caviar sauce
- Buttered peas with mint
- Finger vegetables
- Mung vegetable mold on sprouts
- Vinaigrette
- Carrot juice

EARLY SNACK
- Piima custard with fruit

LATE SNACK
- Apple and almonds

DINNER
- Millet dish
- Tossed green salad
- Bleu cheese dressing
- Dill crock
- Almond milk
- Carrot and beet juice

SNACK
- 14-grain cereal

SECOND DAY

Upon Arising
- Tomato cocktail

BREAKFAST
- Ginger tea
- 14-grain cereal

SNACK
- Carrot juice

LUNCH
- Vegetarian chop suey
- Broccoli
- Hollandaise sauce
- Tossed green salad
- Basic french dressing
- Finger vegetables
- Vinaigrette
- Celery and carrot juice

EARLY SNACK
- Yogurt sundae

LATE SNACK
- Pear and cheese
- Green vegetable juice

DINNER
- Cheese tacos
- Tomato ribbon aspic on sprouts
- Mexican pickles
- Herb tea
- Fruit juice

SNACK
- Blueberry whirl

Please Note: These menus are samples only and do not represent a complete nutritional therapy program. The authors do not advise that anyone use these particular foods in repetition.

(Chapter Addendum)

Extra Information On Diet

"Sample Recipes"

Piima Low-Protein Drink

1 cup Piima yogurt
1 tablespoon lemon or lime juice
1 tablespoon honey

Quickly stir or blend all ingredients together.

Variations: In place of lemon juice, use ⅓ cup of any fresh raw fruit—or ½ cup of any fruit juice except citrus, adding honey. This recipe may be used at any time of the day.

Piima Medium-Protein Drink

2 fertile eggs
1 cup Piima yogurt
1 tablespoon ground almonds
1 tablespoon honey, sorghum or molasses
1 teaspoon vanilla

Blend in blender just long enough to mix.

Variations: Add one or more of the following: 1 tablespoon carob powder and ½ medium banana, or ⅓ cup raw fruit except citrus, or ½ cup fruit juice except citrus. This recipe should be eaten before 3:00 p.m.

Piima Medium Protein Natural Custard

2 cups Piima yogurt
2 fertile eggs
1 teaspoon vanilla
⅛ cup sorghum or molasses, or ¼ cup honey
1 tablespoon Knox or Grayslake gelatin
¼ cup cold water or juice

Soak gelatin in water, then melt over low heat, stirring constantly. Place sorghum, yogurt, vanilla, eggs in the blender. Blend briefly, then add melted gelatin while blender is whirling. Pour into custard cups and sprinkle with nutmeg.

Variations: Add any of the following:

a. ½ medium-size banana and 1 or 2 tablespoons of carob powder;
b. Omit honey and use 5 or 6 pitted dates;
c. For a butterscotch flavor, add ¼ cup fig juice, or reconstituted "Fig Pep" from health food store.

This recipe should be eaten before 3:00 p.m.

Piima Ice Cream, Low Protein

2 cups Piima cream
¼ cup honey
1 or 2 tablespoons grated orange, lemon or tangerine peel
½ cup juice from any of the above fruit

Blend and place in bowl in freezer until frozen to a thick mush. Remove from freezer and beat until smooth. Return to freezer until desired consistency is achieved. Makes 1½ pints.

Sauteed Fish

Pat fish dry with paper towel. Dip in beaten egg and then into a mixture of ⅛ cup bran and ⅛ cup brown rice flour, then place into skillet with melted butter and gently heat until coating is golden on each side—a very few minutes.

Egg Foo Yung

To 4 eggs, beaten with fork, add:

- 1 tablespoon arrowroot flour
- ½ cup mung bean sprouts
- ¼ cup sliced scallions
- ¼ cup snow peas, sliced diagonally
- ¼ cup sliced Jerusalem artichokes
- ¼ cup chopped green pepper
- 2 tablespoons soy sauce

Mix ingredients and cook like pancakes in electric frying pan at the table. Serve additional sauce if desired.

French Carrot Salad

Shred enough carrots (fine) to make a large mound for each person.

For the dressing, mix in blender:

- ½ cup olive oil
- ¼ cup vinegar
- ⅓ teaspoon Dijon-type French mustard
- 1 teaspoon fresh horseradish
- 1 fat clove of garlic, crushed, or a few drops garlic oil
- ¼ teaspoon seasoning salt to taste
- ½ teaspoon ground papaya seeds to taste

This dressing is also delicious on sliced tomatoes or cucumbers. Use less dressing than you think necessary as you toss the shredded carrots, taste, then add more if necessary. Store excess dressing for later salads. Serve on a bed of alfalfa sprouts topped with a mound of the marinated carrots.

Medley Pancakes

3 eggs
½ cup sunflower seeds, ground
½ cup pumpkin or sesame seeds, ground
¼ cup corn, ground
½ cup arrowroot starch
¼ cup wheat bran or rice bran
2 tablespoons butter
½ cup Piima yogurt or water
1 teaspoon sesame salt
1 teaspoon cinnamon
¼ teaspoon nutmeg

Mix all ingredients and bake on buttered griddle or electric skillet at the table. You may choose to add 1 tablespoon honey or the sweetener of your choice to the batter and serve the pancakes with butter only. Or, omit the sweetener and serve with fruit and pit jam and butter.

Almond Milk

Place 1 cup sprouted almonds in blender with ½ cup water and blend until smooth mush, then gradually add up to 3½ cups more water, 1 teaspoon of honey and ¼ teaspoon of barley malt sweetener, plus 1 teaspoon vanilla. You may choose to use part almonds and part sprouted sunflower seeds or sprouted sesame seeds instead of almonds. For cream, use ½ the amount of water. This is an excellent substitution for milk or cream when milk is restricted from your diet. Try making eggnogs or raw custards with seed milks.

Please Note: These recipes are intended as samples only. They are merely healthy foods that can be a part of an individualized nutritional program. These recipes are not intended to be used repetitiously as the only parts of a diet.

CHAPTER TWELVE

The Power of Food Supplements

Physicians who tell their cancer patients that they are receiving enough nutrients from their foods, and need no supplements, are, in the opinions of metabolic physicians, exposing their lack of knowledge about nutrition. Even if the patient's diet is composed of fresh, whole foods, say these doctors, the foods in the diet almost certainly lack sufficient nutrients to help a ravaged body regain health. During the reversal of cancer, they say, the body needs to be flooded with nutrients, more nutrients than one can receive from whole foodstuffs.

Consumption of optimum levels of vitamins, minerals and enzymes is said to not only prevent most cancers, even in persons exposed to high levels of carcinogens, but also to help the body to destroy existing malignancies. These optimum nutrient levels, though, are considered virtually impossible to meet through normal dietary intake, and are considered especially difficult to fulfill in cancer patients, whose nutritional requirements are far more demanding than those of healthy people.

The gradual deterioration of our agricultural and foods resources has made achieving proper nutrition more difficult than ever. "During the past 150 years," maintains Dr. W. C. Hueper of the National Cancer Institute, "man has fundamentally changed and revolutionized the natural environment in which he and animals are living, by the effects of a rapidly increasing industrialization of the human activities, and by the alarmingly growing chemicalization of the environment of man and animals, including their food supply. . . ."[1] Not only is there now an untamed menagerie of chemicals circulating in our environment, which require vast amounts of nutrients to deactivate them, but there is also a scarcity of these badly needed nutrients available from our depleted agri-industry.

Conversion to monoculture (growing only one crop), and heavy use of chemical fertilizers and pesticides, says Charles McGee, M.D., as well as increased hybridization and chemical growth stimulation of animals, has resulted in production of devitalized, degraded food products that may look large, glossy and rich, but are in reality only a few steps above junk food.[2] Dr. McGee indicts as nutrient-depleters: Use of nitrate fertilizers; "mining" of the soil's minerals; breeding of tough, hard food and products that will resist the rigors of machine harvesting and processing; and application of common food storage techniques.

As a result of these agricultural influences, and poor eating habits in general, the U.S. Department of Agriculture now estimates that "48 per cent of all households do not fully meet approved intake of one or more nutrients."[3]

Shopping in health food stores, open-air markets, and at reputable truck gardens, as well as growing one's own food, can help overcome the problem of nutrient depletion. But none of these measures are a panacea. Many stores are "health food" stores more by style than content. And even if one is able to buy or grow nutritious food, the amounts of nutrients needed to compensate for living in our polluted, stressful environment may still not be met. For example, say metabolic doctors, in order to receive sufficient vitamin C, which could range from one to two grams daily for a healthy person who lives in our busy, polluted society—and could be as much as 50 grams in a very ill cancer patient—one would have to eat between 20 and 1000 oranges per day. To get enough potassium, which would be about 300-400 milligrams per day for a healthy, hard working person, and one gram per day for a cancer patient, a healthy person would have to eat ten helpings of raw green beans a day, and a cancer patient would have to eat 30 to 40 helpings.[4] The only way to receive the nutrients that modern life demands, if no supplements are taken, is to juice enormous quantities of fresh fruits and vegetables, a nutrient-condensing tactic that is an expensive, time-consuming proposition. And even enormous amounts of juices, say metabolic doctors, are unlikely to produce enough nutrients to meet the demands of a cancer patient.

People often ask metabolic doctors, "If use of supplements is so necessary, why do some people not take them and remain healthy?" These people, say the doctors, may have exceptionally strong constitutions. They may exercise vigorously. These people are probably not as healthy as they could be if they took supplements, and still may eventually die of cancer, heart disease, or another degenerative disease, as do three out of every four Americans. Consider this: Over 85 per cent of us contract a serious degenerative disease or chronic condition, about 40 per cent of us are obese, and about 95 per cent of us die earlier than do people in societies that live in unpolluted areas and eat only whole, natural foods, such as the Hunzas of Russia.

If the need for supplementation is accepted by most researchers of nutritional science, the need for optimum—rather than minimum—fulfillment of needs is rather less appreciated. The concept of meeting "minimum daily requirements" has two serious shortcomings: (1) it does not adequately allow for individual differences in nutritional needs, and (2) it is based upon waiting for the appearance of obvious physical abnormalities, rather than in recognizing the more subtle signs of gradual deterioration that appear to precede diseases like cancer.

Minimum nutritional requirements at breakfast can be met with a bowl of Chocolate Frosties in milk with a bag of Beer Nuts on the side. Is this really adequate nutrition? The captains of America's food processing industry would like consumers to think so. But, in reality, a daily diet based on these kinds of foods which is, sadly, not far from the norm, affords a scant excess of the nutrients needed to keep one from dropping dead from starvation. A diet like this is not considered sufficient to keep one from contracting cancer or heart disease, and is thought to be hardly enough to fill the nutritional demands of a cancer patient.

The program of optimum nutrition that metabolic doctors apply to cancer patients, which has clear therapeutic effects, involves regular, intensive supplementation with vitamins, minerals, enzymes and extracts of animal glands and organs. The physicians recommend supplementation before, during and after each meal, in the afternoons, before bedtime, and often in the middle of the night. Eating supplements with meals naturally complements the nutrients in foods, and aids digestion, absorption and assimilation. Supplementation is heavier in the first stages of the program, and is gradually reduced as health returns.

There are said to be several benefits of supplementation, which is, of course, part and parcel of the entire nutritional therapy component of a metabolic program. These benefits include: strengthening natural immunity to cancer; deactivating carcinogens and toxins created by tumors; retarding tumor growth; directly attacking tumor masses; and strengthening general systemic function.

All of these functions are of the utmost importance. Without the benefit derived from supplements, metabolic doctors say, these functions would be essentially impossible to achieve, and many more patients would fail in their struggles to recover.

Strengthening Immunity

Vitamin C has a powerful stimulating effect upon the immune mechanisms that kill cancer cells. The immune system, the most important part of which is the cancer-killing white blood cells, is directly dependent upon the body's nutrient intake, and particularly its supply of vitamin C.

Cancer-killing antibodies, which travel in the blood and are found in cells, are in greater evidence in people with higher levels of vitamin C. This was proven by S. Vallance in 1977, who studied subjects who were isolated in Antarctica for a year.[5] The same phenomenon was observed in guinea pigs by Dr. George Feigen of Stanford University.[6] Dr. Feigen also showed that vitamin C was necessary to produce "C_1 esterase," which helps the immune system identify cancer cells as being foreign invaders.[7]

In 1976 National Cancer Institute researchers Chretien and Yonemoto proved that vitamin C increases production of lymphocytes, white blood corpuscles that destroy cancer cells. They found that five grams daily intake produced a noticeable increase in lymphocyte production, and that ten grams resulted in even greater production.[8] They also found that vitamin C* intake increased "blastogenesis," or production of lymphocyte cells by budding.[9]

In 1979 Montreal researchers showed that several nutrients, including vitamin C, linoleic acid, gammalinoleic acid, zinc and pyridoxine, increased a substance that is needed for manufacture of T-lymphocytes, which help the body identify cancer cells.

"The simplest and safest way to enhance immunocompetence" in cancer patients, says Dr. Linus Pauling, "is to increase their intake of vitamin C."[10]

Vitamin C also stimulates activity of Interferon, the natural anti-cancer agent that scientists are now trying to synthesize. The concept that vitamin C increases Interferon was proven by Siegel in 1974 and Schwerdt in 1975.[11]

Dr. A. E. Axelrod of the Pittsburg University Medical School believes that vitamins B_6, folic acid and pantothenic acid are of crucial importance in the immune system's response to cancer. He has said that "no circulatory antibodies whatsoever can be produced in the absence of these specific factors."[12] Dr. Paul Newberne of MIT agrees with Axelrod on the importance of these B vitamins to the immune system, and believes that choline and B_{12}, as well as the amino acid methionine, are also extremely important in maintaining natural immunity to cancer and other diseases.

Nobel Prize winner Otto Warburg has stated that vitamins B_2, B_3 and pantothenic acid are vital in stimulating the immune responses to cancer. He has said that these vitamins are necessary to produce certain enzymes that are important to the immune system.[13]

Deactivating Carcinogens

To recover from cancer, say metabolic doctors, the impact of cancer-causing agents must be avoided. The body frequently does not have sufficient strength to overcome malignancy, they say, if it is simultaneously having to deactivate new toxic substances that are being introduced into it. In this "sea of carcinogens" that we have created as our chosen environment, it is necessary to deflect the inevitable bombardment of cancer-causing agents with deactivating nutrients. Vitamins C, A and E, the mineral selenium and some enzymes can deactivate carcinogens.

"Vitamin C," says Dr. Richard Passwater, "protects us against some cancer-causing chemicals, such as nitrites, and directly detoxifies still other carcinogens."[14] Dr. Sidney Mirvish of the University of Nebraska Medical Center showed that vitamin C blocked in the stomach the conversion of nitrites into nitrosamines, which are the form of the compound that causes cancer.[15]

Vitamin C has also been shown, as long ago as 1930, to destroy the carcinogens benzopyrene and acetaldehyde, two of the most lethal cancer-causers in cigarette smoke.[16]

Vitamin C in the urine interferes with the conversion of 3-hydroxyanthranilic acid to cinnabaric acid, a substance that is closely related to incidence of bladder cancer.[17] It is hypothesized that the high incidence of bladder cancer in smokers is due to the displacement of vitamin C in having to destroy the toxins in cigarette smoke.[18]

Dr. W. Robert Bruce, of the University of Toronto, announced in 1977 his belief that 75 per cent of the potential cancer-causing agents in the common industrialized diet could be deactivated in the bowel by the presence of vitamin C.[19]

"It is likely," wrote Linus Pauling in *Vitamin C and Cancer,* "that part of the effectiveness of vitamin C in helping to decrease cancer results from its power to act as a rather general detoxifying agent. In collaboration with molecular oxygen and certain enzymes in the human body, it converts toxic substances, including those that cause cancer, into non-toxic derivatives that then are eliminated in the urine."[20]

Vitamin C is not the only nutrient that deactivates toxins. Arthur Upton, M.D., former Director of the National Cancer Institute, told a recent Senate Hearing that many nutritional factors blunted the carcinogenic effect of many of the most common cancer-causers. "An enzyme system called the microsomal mixed-function oxidase system," he said, "appears to exert a protective effect in detoxifying carcinogens."[21] Dr. Upton also named selenium, and vitamins C and E and A, as having "a protective effect against chemical carcinogenesis."[22]

A report from the Diet, Nutrition and Cancer program of the National Cancer Institute said that "high intakes of vitamin A have been shown to reduce chemical carcinogenesis in epithelial cells and to depress gastric tumor growth."[23]

Drs. Donald Hill and Tzu-Wen Shih said in 1974 that they believed vitamin A prohibits intermediate compounds in the body that normally result from exposure to carcinogens.[24] David Kaufman of the National Cancer Institute also showed in 1974 that carcinogens bind more tightly to DNA from vitamin A deficient animals, thus increasing their chances of malignant cell formation.[25] Dr. Curtis Port of the Illinois Institute of Technology recently reported that vitamin A reduced lung cancer in animals repeatedly exposed to carcinogens.[26]

Vitamin E is also an excellent detoxifying agent. Vitamin E, which is an antioxidant, has been proven capable of nullifying the harmful irradiation of excessive exposure to the sun, which causes skin cancer.[27] A 1972 article in the *Journal of Agriculture and Food Chemistry* said that rats given extra vitamin E were able to withstand the effects of various pollutants 50 to 100 per cent longer than rats deficient in vitamin E.[28] In an experiment reported in the *Proceedings of the National Academy of Sciences,* researchers at the Cleveland Clinic Foundation found that vitamin E, when applied to cells that had been exposed to carcinogens, decreased cellular damage by 63.2 per cent, compared to cells with no extra protective nutrients.

Selenium is also a good detoxifier. Also an antioxidant, it showed an ability in the Cleveland Clinic test to halt chromosomal damage due to carcinogen exposure even more effectively than vitamin C.

Some enzymes detoxify. "A particular kind of enzyme in rats," writes Donald Germann, M.D., "detoxifies carcinogenic substances administered to the animals."[29]

It is our belief, based upon clinical observation, that these detoxifying agents are also effective in deactivating the toxins produced by tumors. Cancer has been shown by many researchers to exude toxic substances into the bloodstream, and it has become apparent that destroyed malignant cells produce even more toxic stress upon the body while they are being discharged through the organs of elimination.

For the healthy person, use of detoxifying supplements is an excellent way of preventing cancer. For the cancer patient, these detoxifiers are an indispensable means of regaining health. These poison-neutralizing agents free the body's own "invader-killing" forces to wage a war against cancer.

Protecting Healthy Cells

Nutrients also protect malignant cells' healthy "neighbors" from "invasion." Vitamin C is particularly adept at this function. Cancer cells produce an enzyme, hyaluronidase, which breaks down the intercellular material that protects healthy cells, rendering these cells vulnerable to the malignant process. Vitamin C, Dr. Ewan Cameron showed in the late 1960s, strengthens the intercellular material that hyaluronidase attacks.[30] Dr. Linus Pauling, who collaborated with Dr. Cameron, writes, "The fortunate patient with a good supply of vitamin C may develop a very slowly growing, practically non-invasive tumor, encased in a dense, almost impermeable barrier of scar tissue, giving him a clinical prognosis differing little from normal life expectancy."[31] Because of the strengthening of resistance of healthy cells, vitamin C was shown by Dr. Cameron to markedly decrease cancer patients' pain, which is frequently associated with initial invasion of new cells.[32]

Vitamin A is another nutrient that helps protect healthy cells from malignancy. Dr. George Plotkin of M.I.T. said that, "A deficiency of vitamin A prevents a mucous coating from forming on the trachea, lungs, rectum, digestive system and on the inside of the skin. The vitamin A deficiency doesn't cause cancer, but it makes these areas less able to resist cancer.[33]

Dr. Michael Sporn of the National Cancer Institute has said that, "Well over half of all human cancer starts in epithelial tissue, the tissue that forms the lining of organs, forms glands, such as mammary glands, and forms skin and passages in the body. The respiratory tract, the digestive tract, the urinary tract and the reproductive tract are all lined with epithelial tissue. And all of the specialized cells that form epithelial tissue depend on vitamin A for their normal development." Dr. Umberyo Saffoti and his collaborators, said Dr. Sporn, "showed that vitamin A had some ability to protect animals from development of lung cancer ten years ago. . . ."[34]

Vitamin E, which strengthens the cell membranes of every cell in the body, is also needed to help healthy cells resist the onslaught of malignancy.

Direct Anti-Tumoral Activities

Some nutrients appear to have direct impact upon tumors. Vitamins A and B appear to interfere with the process of malignant cell growth, and certain pancreatic enzymes have repeatedly shown a superb ability to directly attack the cell walls of malignant masses.

Retinoids, which are compounds very similar to vitamin A, were called by the N.C.I.'s Dr. Sporn, "hormone-like controllers of cell differentiation."[35] Dr. Sporn said that adequate amounts of vitamin A encourage cells to stay in a mature differentiated state, rather than to revert to the undifferentiated condition characteristic of malignant cells. "Whether this actually arrests the process of development of cancer or whether this causes the precancerous cells to disappear from tissue is a topic of current research," he said.[36]

Dr. Raymond Shamberger of the Cleveland Clinic concluded, after a series of experiments, that "Vitamin A retards the growth and inhibits induction of benign and malignant tumors."[37] It is theorized by Dr. Otto Warburg and others that all of the anti-oxidative nutrients, including vitamins A and E and the mineral selenium, interfere with the respiration of malignant cells.

U.C.L.A. research recently revealed that vitamin B_3, when added to laboratory cultures of cancer cells, inhibited the abnormal protein synthesis of the cancer cells, thereby retarding their growth.[38]

Virtually all holistic cancer therapists, including those who work with Dr. W. D. Kelley, have seen much clinical evidence of enzymes helping to break down fully-developed, often metastasized tumors, through a mechanism of action presumed to be that of dissolving the wall of malignant cells, thereby enabling the white blood cells of the immune system to kill the malignant cells. Enzymes have a more noticeable effect than any of the other supplements often administered in metabolic programs. Cancer therapists who use copious doses of enzymes have repeatedly said that cancer is most aptly characterized as an enzyme deficiency disease. The pancreatic enzymes trypsin and chymotrypsin appear to be especially effective in helping to break down tumor masses.

The special ability of enzymes to break down cancer cell walls was noted as long ago as 1888, when the enzyme pepsin was applied directly to ulcerated cancer lesions. Over the years, researchers and therapists, including Dr. John Beard, of Scotland, and Dr. E. Freund, of Austria, refined enzyme treatment of cancer, determining that the protein-digesting enzymes seemed to be of the most value against malignancy, presumably because the tough cell wall of a cancer cell is partially formed of protein.[39]

By the early 1960s, extensive tests had shown that tumors did respond to enzyme application. In a study of over 1000 cancer patients treated with enzymes and radiotherapy at the Wolf-Zimmer Clinic in Germany, it was determined that between 65.1 per cent and 68 per cent of the patients studied achieved objective improvement of condition.[40] This improvement rate was much higher than that commonly achieved at that time with only radiotherapy. At that same clinic, according to Max Wolf, M.D. and Karl Ransberger, Ph.D., authors of *Enzyme Therapy,* over 13,000 cancer patients were treated with enzymes.[41]

More recent studies of enzyme use for cancer have been conducted by researcher R. Titscher, of the University of Vienna, who noted considerable improvement in cancer patients who were treated with enzymes.[42] In a four-year study concluded in 1972, Titscher found that an enzyme concentration used against tumors was a more effective anti-tumoral agent than any of several other more commonly used agents that he had experimented with.[43]

European cancer researcher Dr. Hoefer-Janker also recently reported similarly positive results with enzyme therapy.[44]

Harold Manner, Ph.D., extensively studied the reactions of tumors to enzyme therapy throughout the 1970s. He wrote in the late 1970s of his strong belief that enzymes enable the tough cancer cell wall to be penetrated by natural immune forces. "Clinics around the world are using digestive enzyme complexes in conjunction with irradiation, chemotherapy, surgery and nutritional therapies. . . ." he wrote in *The Death of Cancer*. "The enzyme treatment makes sense, is a natural approach, and has had positive results."[45]

There are several reasons for the possible existence of an enzyme insufficiency in a patient's body. The pancreas may be dysfunctional to the degree that it fails to produce sufficient enzymes. Enzymes may be diverted by large amounts of protein ingested as part of the diet. There may be a lack of vitamins or minerals which are "co-enzymes" (the catalysts needed for enzymes to fulfill their functions). There may be too many anti-enzyme factors impinging upon the body, such as toxic substances in the diet or environment. There may be an inadequate supply of blood to carry the enzymes to the site of malignancy. There may be a failure of the systems that metabolize vitamins and minerals, without which enzymes cannot complete their full chemical processes. Any of these various factors can result in an insufficient supply of pancreatic enzymes, and can, according to metabolic doctors, be the major predisposing factor to onset of malignancy. Most of these inhibitory factors can also contribute to creation of the other inhibitory factors, creating a downward cycle of enzymatic function.

Lack of enzymes, by disrupting digestive and assimilative function, can cause systemic failure and general loss of energy. This is the final way that lack of specific nutrients can negatively affect malignancy. Every organ in the body helps in some way to fight cancer, and the liver, pancreas, kidneys, stomach, colon, and other organs play extremely important roles in resistance to malignancy. Supplementation can greatly stimulate the function of these organs, both by supplying their tissues with the needed nutrients and by partially substituting for their function. The B vitamins, for example, are of paramount importance in insuring adequate liver function, and proper liver function is considered an absolute necessity in a patient's fight against cancer. Vitamin C also can help the liver, by neutralizing some of the toxins that would otherwise have gone to the liver for detoxification.

With cancer, as with other diseases, there is often a temptation to focus upon the disease's most specific symptoms, which are often confined to single organs and systems, rather than to consider all of the organs and systems. Many presumably "holistic" cancer therapists recommend supplements that will impact primarily upon the tumor mass, or perhaps upon the tumor and certain obviously-related organs, such as the pancreas or liver. This segmented, isolationist approach characterizes mechanistic medicine, and is generally a detriment to healing. To rid itself of tumors, say metabolic doctors, the body not only needs enzymes from the pancreas, but also blood from the heart, oxygen from the lungs, nutrients from the stomach, and agents from the lymphatic system. If each of the organs governing these components is not functioning well, they say, healing will be impaired. Supplementation with mega-nutrients, according to metabolic physicians, is one of the most effective ways to insure proper function of all of these important components of health, and should not be directed at just the tumor and one or two other organs.

A Daily Supplemental Regime

The first supplements of the day for a cancer patient under the care of a metabolic doctor are taken at about 3:30 a.m., when the body reaches its daily peak of alkalinity, and cell walls are most permeable to influx of nutrients and egress of toxins. At this time, ten pancreatic enzyme tablets are taken, which contain, among other enzymes, trypsin and chymotrypsin, which seem especially effective in breaking through the tough malignant cell walls.

All supplements may be taken with pure, preferably distilled water, or with juice. Many people prefer to use juice, since their nutritional program requires drinking such large amounts of it. For those who have difficulty in swallowing pills, some of the supplements may be chewed or ground up. Because the taste of some of the supplements may be objectionable, they may be mixed with juice after grinding. Grinding or chewing some tablets helps in the digestion of them.

About half an hour before breakfast, patients take their first before-meal supplements. Supplements are taken before, during and after each meal. The before-meal supplements are often minerals and glandular or organ extracts.

Glandular and organ extracts, or "protomorphogens," are

animal glands that are believed to stimulate and support the corresponding gland or organ in the person that ingests them. They have the amino acids, nutrients, and RNA and DNA molecules, all in the proper proportion, that are needed by that particular human organ or gland. Radioimmunoassay tests have shown that these "organ specific biological activators" are taken up by the phagocytes in the blood and carried directly to the corresponding human organ or gland.[46] Of special importance to the cancer patient is stimulation with protomorphogens of the thymus (an important part of the immune system), the liver, the pituitary (the endocrine system's "master regulator"), the toxin-draining lymphatic glands, and often the particular organ or glandular site of malignancy.

Enzymes are eaten during every meal, to help aid digestion. Vitamins and minerals are taken directly after meals, to synergize the nutrient content of the meals.

Enzymes are also eaten in the mid-afternoon, when the body again reaches its apogee of alkalinity.

Prior to bedtime, many patients take some calming supplements, such as calcium or tryptophan or magnesium, in order to sleep better.

Cycling Enzymes

Because supplementation with pancreatic enzymes seems to have such a powerful, direct anti-tumoral action, enzyme supplementation appears to sometimes be able to help the patient kill malignant cells faster than the patient can eliminate them. When this happens, the organs of elimination, particularly the liver, are unable to discharge all the toxins that accumulate in the system, causing "toxic" symptoms, similar to those of influenza, such as nausea, chills, loss of appetite and energy, headache, fever and lymphatic swelling. These symptoms, which are generally characterized as "healing crises," can usually be overcome by discontinuing enzyme use and increasing detoxification measures. If not properly responded to, say metabolic doctors, this reaction to tumor breakdown can result in symptoms of severe toxicity and even death. Most people who have solid tumor masses are advised to use enzyme supplementation in cycles.

Cycling of enzymes in an on/off pattern is easily accomplished. Most people can begin their program of supplementation, including use of enzymes, for 10 to 21 days without a toxic reaction. When the first toxic "healing crisis" occurs, signaling necrotic tumor-debris build-up in the eliminative organs, it can be countered with a five-day discontinuation of supplements. The cycling schedule is adjusted for each patient, based upon the degree of his or her toxic reaction. The more overt the toxic symptoms, the longer the person should remain in the off-cycle. Some people can only take the supplements for a few days without becoming ill.

Because use of the supplements, especially the enzymes, seems to facilitate tumor destruction, a person with cancer is advised to stay on the on-cycle as long as possible and the off-cycle for as short a time as possible, within the boundaries of comfort and general health. Five days is the maximum length of time in the off-cycle for a seriously ill person. People are advised to attempt to reach the first stages of toxicity without becoming "dragged down" by toxic reactions. Supplements, according to metabolic doctors, should not be taken for so long that pronounced toxic symptoms, such as vomiting or total appetite loss, appear.

As one recovers, he or she will begin to require a shorter off-cycle period because less tumor mass is being excreted by the system.

Of special value, according to metabolic doctors, for feelings of toxicity brought on by tumor breakdown is the coffee enema, explained in detail in the following chapter. This procedure stimulates liver function and curtails many toxic symptoms. If one's toxic reaction to supplementation is severe, as many as two to three coffee enemas per day may be indicated.

Results of Supplementation

Literally hundreds of studies, tests and experiments have been made on the relationship between recovery from cancer and hyperalimentation with food supplements. Virtually all of them have shown that mega-nutrition with food supplements is a valuable component of a cancer therapy program. The following represent a cross-section of all the research that has been done.

One of the more dramatic human studies was done with vitamin C, under the direction of Dr. Ewan Cameron of Vale of Lebanon Hospital in Scotland, and Dr. Linus Pauling. In 1976 they compared survival statistics of 100 terminally ill patients given 10 grams (10,000 milligrams) of vitamin C per day, and those of 1000 terminally ill patients not given vitamin C. Other than use of vitamin C, there were no other appreciable differences in the patients' treatments. The patients given vitamin C lived an average of four times longer than the other patients. Sixteen of the 100 vitamin C patients lived over one year, compared to three of the 1000 other patients. Twelve of the 100 vitamin C patients, or 12 per cent, completely recovered from cancer, while all 1000 of the others died. The patients treated with vitamin C also showed improved quality of life, including less pain and a better appetite; five patients on heavy morphine schedules were able to be taken off all pain-relieving drugs.[47]

Dr. Pauling stated that he felt higher recovery rates could have been achieved with higher doses of the vitamin. Dr. Pauling believes that approximately 10 grams of vitamin C per day is a proper dose for a healthy person and insufficient for a cancer patient.[48] Vitamin C researcher Dr. Irwin Stone recommends 50 grams daily for cancer patients. In 1977 Dr. Pauling said, "With proper use of vitamin C for cancer, we could cut the death rate by 75 per cent."[49]

Large population studies support the efficacy of vitamin C use for cancer patients. Drs. Chope and Breslow found in an eight-year study of San Mateo County residents that those with the higher consumptions of vitamin C had approximately one-half the cancer death rate of those with lower consumptions.[50] In 1973 Norwegian researcher Dr. E. Bjelke surveyed 30,000 people and found that the greater their regular ingestion of vitamin C, the less common was their incidence of cancer.[51]

Dr. Bjelke also studied the epidemiological relationship between use of vitamin A and cancer incidence. In a five-year study of 8,278 male smokers, he found that 74 per cent of men with lung cancer were in the lowest one-third of his group in vitamin A intake. He also found that vitamin A deficient city dwellers had 300 per cent more lung cancer than those who had sufficient vitamin A intake.[52]

In 1976 Dr. Bernard P. Lane of New York State University exposed tissues from 200 tracheae for three weeks to a cancer-causing agent. He found that he could reverse the carcinogenic effects of the cancer-causing agent by treating the tissue samples with vitamin A.[53] Also in 1976, Dr. Alex Sakula of Rehill General Hospital in England found that blood levels of vitamin A were lower than normal in all 28 of his bronchial cancer patients.[54]

Drs. Cheraskin, Ringsdorf and Clark report in *Diet and Disease* that four human experiments on the cancer leukoplakia showed inhibition of leukoplakia tumors in the presence of large doses of vitamin A. In one double-blind controlled experiment, 400,000 I.U. of vitamin A taken each day for 21 days resulted in "a reduction in size, favorable qualitative change in the lesions, and histiologic evidence of improvement in a substantial sample of the vitamin A supplemental group."[55]

B vitamins were shown therapeutically effective for the cancer neuroblastoma by Dr. M. Bodian in 1963.[56] In an experiment reported in the *Journal of Nutrition,* Dr. Kanematsu Sugiura, lately of Sloan-Kettering, exposed 100 rats to carcinogens, but gave 50 of them high doses of B vitamins. The 50 rats with B vitamins remained 30 per cent cancer-free, while all 50 of those without B vitamins died from cancer.[57]

In a human experiment reported in the *Journal of Urology,* the B vitamin inositol, given to six bladder cancer patients, reduced the size of their tumors and stopped blood from appearing in their urine.[58] Canadian urologist Dr. Balfour Mount of McGill University has found vitamin B_6 helpful for treating bladder cancer patients.[59]

Selenium was shown to be linked to resistance to malignancy in a test of 1000 patients done by Dr. John Martin of Colorado State University. Dr. Martin told *Prevention* magazine, "The results were startling. There was a positive inverse relationship between cancer involvement and serum selenium."[60]

Whole Food Supplements

The use of these various nutrients is obviously highly valuable. However, many metabolic and immunologic cancer therapists are, the author feels, incorrectly using isolated vitamins and minerals. When they use these nutrients pharmacologically, either in isolated, single-nutrient applications, or in limited mixtures of two or three nutrients, the doctors fail to get the most possible good from the nutrients. Very prudent patients employ not only a wide range of supplements, but also supplements that are comprised of whole-foods products, rather than isolated, specific nutrients.

Providing nutrients to patients in as complete a form as possible is necessary in order to give the patient all the synergistic, complementary benefits from the various nutrients. It is known that vitamins need the presence of minerals in order to fulfill their functions, and that many enzymes need the presence of vitamins, and vice versa.

It is also known that the body, when confronted with a systemic pathology such as cancer, requires the proper function of virtually all of its major organs and glands and systems to metabolically reverse the disease. It is further known that each of these organs, glands and systems requires varying nutrients.

Adding to the necessity of using whole-food supplements is the fact that nutritional scientists simply do not know all of the various isolated nutrients that are vital for life. Nutrients that are essential for life are classified as vitamins, and the list of necessary vitamins has grown longer and longer as more discoveries have been made.

Dr. William Holub, a professor of nutrition at C.W. Post College, has studied the problems inherent in using isolated vitamins and minerals. Dr. Holub has written that, "If one examines the history of the 'discoveries' of the essentiality of vitamins and minerals, it can be appreciated that the discoveries were made in a context of the "state of the art" of technology at the time. The ability to isolate and describe a need for a nutrient depends on the extent to which our technology can isolate it from a complex food source and then demonstrate its essentiality in an even more complex organism, like man. The histories of the discoveries of the B vitamins document the fact that vitamins are actually complex combinations of many factors, only some of which may be readily isolated. Just when researchers thought there was one B vitamin, they found two:

B_1 and B_2. Inability to correct all of the symptoms of deficiency led to the realization that deficiencies were multi-factorial and did not represent a single vitamin deficiency. Many other factors were subsequently described as members of the B complex group. Currently there is considerable dispute over exactly how many of the B complex vitamins have been 'discovered.'

"Theoretically, as our technical knowledge increases, more and more vitamins and minerals may be uncovered, until some day one may walk into a pharmacy and find 1000 individual nutrients. Knowing, however, which ones and how much of each to take, in order to properly build one's body, will be like trying to rebuild a leaf from its essential elements. While isolation of vitamins and minerals is useful in expanding our understanding of human function, it should not provide the format for dietary requirements.

"To build and sustain health, one must use whole foods and whole food supplements as a daily dietary resource. Whole food supplements are concentrated whole foods known to contain many nutrients, and that have had water and inert material removed. They should be as close to living as possible and contain all the required nutrients and co-factors."

Dr. Holub presents several reasons why whole-food supplements are necessary. They include the following:

1. "Synthetic and isolated vitamins are not absorbed, assimilated and utilized as effectively as they are when they are in their natural state.

2. "Most minerals are not absorbed and utilized properly if not found in association with certain other minerals, molecules and vitamins.

3. "No one knows exactly what amounts and what mixtures of isolated vitamins and minerals stimulate health.

4. "Whole food supplements provide all of the known and as yet unknown vitamins, minerals and other factors we need, in the structures and amounts which our digestive systems have evolved to use.

5. "Our body's nutrient metabolism is like a huge complex mobile. A little weight added to any arm or string can distort the shape of the entire mobile. Introducing isolated nutrients can have this same unbalancing effect on nutrient equilibrium.

6. "Individual vitamins and minerals have pharmacologic action, like a drug, and will stimulate or activate certain segments of metabolism. Thus, while vitamin/mineral therapy may reduce or create symptoms, it is not improving systemic health to its optimum level. Only whole foods and whole food supplements can do that."[61]

Patients on metabolic programs are advised to take as many whole-food supplements, rather than isolated vitamins or minerals, as possible. Among the whole-food supplements recommended are brewer's yeast, rather than synthetic B vitamins; wheat germ oil, rather than synthetic vitamin E; cod liver oil, rather than synthetic vitamin A; concentrated rose hips, rather than synthetic vitamin C; bone meal, rather than synthetic vitamin D; raw liver concentrate, rather than isolated iron; etc. The very best-quality vitamins, minerals, enzymes and protomorphogens are compounded with other nutrient factors. It is not at all unusual for a single high-quality tablet or capsule to contain 10 to 20 nutrients. The clinical experiences of many metabolic doctors and nutritionists have shown that these multi-factorial supplements are extremely effective.

When whole-food products are used, those who take them often have to take larger numbers of tablets or capsules than they would if the supplements were isolated, synthetic products. It might take several brewer's yeast capsules, for example, to equal the number of milligrams of the various B vitamins found in a synthetic brand. Consequently, a person beginning a metabolic program might be advised to take as many as 100 to 200 supplements per day in the first six to 12 months of the program. Fewer supplements could be taken, of course, if synthetic supplements were used, but losing the cofactors found in whole-food supplements could be a serious mistake for a very ill person. Unfortunately, the higher the number of supplements taken, the more the person taking the supplements will have to spend on them. This expense does not, of course, begin to compare to the enormous expenses entailed in the treatments of surgery, radiation or chemotherapy. As a person recovers, supplementation is reduced, thereby reducing the expense.

Unreliability of Brands

One should not be naive enough to think that, just because a corporation is engaged in the manufacture of health products, that it is therefore, in all instances, an altruistic, or even reputable, concern. Many times during recent years, legal action has been taken against supplement companies that have cynically adulterated and weakened their products, to the obvious detriment of their customers. It is not particularly difficult to tamper with the formula of a supplement and escape legal retribution or even public notice. Former F.D.A. commissioner James Goddard recently estimated that consumers spend as much as "$500 million annually" on falsely represented supplements and health products.[62]

One of the more blatant examples of this misrepresentation was the marketing of "Carter's Little Liver Pills." The pills, according to Dr. Murray Katz, "contained absolutely nothing that was good for the liver."[63] Nonetheless, it took the F.D.A. 16 years of litigation to have the word "liver" removed from the pills' label.

People buying supplements should try to base their supplement purchase on the criterion of quality. Those who do not do this generally do not fare as well during a metabolic program as those who purchase the best products available.

Supplements Are Not a Panacea

Hardly a week goes by without the grocery-store checkout-line tabloids affronting us with a headline screaming out "Cancer Cured With Vitamin Z!!" This manipulation of the public consciousness is as crass as it is unbelievable. No individual supplement will ever cure cancer, because the disease is simply too complex to be conquered by a simplistic, single-factor supplement.

There appears to be no magical combination of supplements that will, in and of itself, cure cancer. The public sometimes seems to practically demand that doctors or the news media tell them of such a wondrous "secret formula," though, so inundated are they in the pharmacological "magic bullet" philosophy.

Recovery from cancer, say metabolic physicians, is based upon much more than food supplementation. It is, they say, based upon rigorous, disciplined adherence to a multi-faceted metabolic program for many months, and sometimes years.

Supplementation, however, should not be underestimated. Without this powerful tool, metabolic doctors say, it is less than likely that any person with an advanced cancer would ever be able to recover by using a metabolic program.

Certain specific nutrients such as vitamin A may be toxic if taken in excess. People are advised by the author to check with their physicians prior to ingesting high doses of vitamins and minerals.

CHAPTER THIRTEEN

The Importance of Detoxification

Anyone who has lived the mainstream American lifestyle for ten or more years has 70 trillion garbage cans for cells," says Dwight McKee, M.D., Medical Director of the International Health Institute. Dr. McKee believes that most of the body's approximately 70 trillion cells are jammed with metabolic and environmental toxins accumulated through years of lifestyle abuse and exposure to poisonous chemicals. This condition, say metabolic doctors, is almost certain to exist in cancer patients, whose organs of detoxification and elimination have obviously failed to accomplish one of their most essential tasks—helping to deactivate and eject from the body malignant cells and malignancy-causing chemicals.

Detoxification, or internal cleansing of the body, is considered an absolutely vital element of a metabolic program. Various methods of systemic purification are said to pave the way for the recovery of people with cancer. Without diligent and vigorous participation in these detoxification procedures, say metabolic doctors, a great many people with cancer would simply not recover. Virtually all of the more sophisticated, whole-body therapies for cancer include, as an integral facet of their treatment, a program of applied detoxification.

Metabolic programs stimulate the organs of elimination with a variety of techniques, among them liver and gall bladder flushes, coffee enemas, colonic irrigations, controlled sweating, purges, fasts, kidney and lung stimulation, dry skin brushing, and various forms of bathing. These techniques stimulate the primary organs of detoxification and elimination, which are the liver, kidneys, colon, lungs and skin.

These procedures speed egress of toxins that have built up over many years. Some of these toxins are in the organs of elimination, but most are still in almost every cell in the body. When the organs of elimination are saturated with toxins, say metabolic doctors, toxins in the cells tend to remain in the cells, until the eliminative pathways are "cleared." It is entirely likely, they say, that some of these toxins have directly created or contributed to the malignant condition, either as carcinogenic, chromosome-mutating agents, or as agents that interfere with normal cell metabolism, or as agents that burden the immune-related organs of the body which protect against cancer.

The detoxifying procedures also are said to aid in the discharge of dead malignant cells and other dysfunctional cells that metabolic programs have helped to kill. Dead tumor cells, in particular, pose a threat to the body. They can, in fact, cause a toxic overload so great that death can result. Almost any serious health-stimulating program, say metabolic doctors, will accelerate the normal rate of cell "turnover," thereby necessitating a corresponding increase in rate of dead-cell elimination.

The average person, who considers himself or herself healthy, would probably benefit noticeably from using these techniques. Healthy people who engage in them often report a surge of energy, well-being and resistance to minor ills after detoxification. People with cancer, though, usually say they feel immeasurably better after engaging in detoxifying procedures, sometimes better than they have in years. They are much more likely to recover, according to metabolic physicians, if fully and regularly detoxified.

"Detoxification," writes Robert Bradford in *Now That You Have Cancer,* "means ridding yourself of poisons. Some of the poisons are the result of abnormal and unusual chemical processes in the body. . . . Other poisons have been directly brought in by the air you breathe, the water you drink, and as chemical additives in the food you eat. As a basic part of cancer management, you need to be detoxified."[1]

Avoiding Toxins

Detoxifying can be largely negated by exposure to further

toxins. Various nutrients, as was shown in the two prior chapters, can deactivate the toxic substances in many foods and chemicals, but sole reliance upon biochemical detoxification is thought to be unwise. Large amounts of toxins penetrate this line of defense, and become lodged in the cells and in the organs of elimination.

Thus, cancer patients are advised to minimize exposure to poisonous agents that are found in the workplace, home, air, food and water. Toxins in food and water were discussed in the chapter on diet and cancer, and the toxins in the air, home and workplace were outlined in the chapter "What Really Causes Cancer."

In the opinions of metabolic physicians, the environment a great many of us live in is not conducive to recovery from cancer, because of the extra stress the toxins in that environment place upon our cells and organs of elimination.

Our food is polluted. The average person eats over 75 mg. of food coloring each day.[2] There are 84 different chemicals in just "apple flavor."[3] There are almost a hundred different toxic chemicals that are sprayed on fruit, many of which can cause cancer.[4] Our air is polluted. Cancer rates soar in not only heavily-polluted urban areas but also remote towns clustered around smelters and small factories.[5] Our water is polluted. In a major government study of 79 of the country's largest water systems, all 79 were found to contain significant quantities of cancer-causing substances.[6] Our water-supplying rivers are filled with coal tar, pitch, oil, dye and rubber wastes, and plastics.[7] Our workplaces are polluted. The federal government recently indicated that as many as 40 per cent of all cancers may stem from workplace pollutants.[8] Even our homes are polluted. Charles McGee, M.D., has shown that the average American home, filled with synthetic products, poisons, and chemical agents, is often more polluted than the environment outside the home.[9]

It is the responsibility of individuals to remove themselves from exposure to these toxins. The toxins most easily avoided are those in our "micro-environment"—composed of the water and food we ingest, the homes we live in, and the cigarettes we smoke. One has total control over one's personal habits and home furnishings. Changing articles in the home to natural wood and fiber products, avoiding cigarettes, and using organic cleaning materials and cosmetics is not very difficult. It is somewhat harder to change our "macro-environment," composed of the air we breathe, and the radiation levels and outdoor and job-site chemicals we are exposed to. One can generally only remove oneself from an unhealthy city or job, as opposed to transforming the city or job-site. But even moving to a new area or finding a new job can be done without severely disrupting one's life. Many cancer patients on metabolic programs have done this.

The sacrifices entailed in changing one's micro- and macro-environment may seem onerous, but are not so unbearable when compared to the possibility of not recovering. Continued exposure to toxic agents can, according to metabolic doctors, frustrate a patient's attempts to detoxify, and can result in disastrous consequences.

The Importance of Detoxifying the Liver and Gall Bladder

Of all the important organs of detoxification and elimination, metabolic physicians believe that the liver is the most important. It is no coincidence, they think, that liver cancer has one of the highest death rates of any cancer when treated with chemotherapy or radiation—without a functioning liver, one not further stressed by an invasive therapy, a cancer patient has little chance of recovery.

The liver, which works in conjunction with the gall bladder, is an incredibly complex organ, the body's largest, and performs thousands of tasks, not all of which physicians even know about. Among its most important functions are:

1. Metabolizing essential fats (cholesterol, triglycerides, lipoproteins) and thus preventing their accumulation in the bloodstream, where they often form deposits on blood vessel walls (atherosclerosis).

2. Synthesizing the bulk of necessary blood proteins.

3. Breaking down and eliminating toxic substances.

4. Secreting a fluid (bile) which is stored in the gall bladder or the enlarged bile duct and empties into the small intestine. This bile acts as a carrier for all liver wastes. It is also essential

for the proper digestion and assimilation of fats and all fat-soluble nutrients, such as vitamins A, D, E, K, lecithin, and the essential fatty acids.

The gall bladder is a hollow muscular organ which stores and concentrates bile, and is attached to the undersurface of the liver. When a meal is eaten, especially one containing some fats or oils, the gall bladder is stimulated to contract. It should freely expel its contents into the small intestine to emulsify fatty nutrients for proper absorption. It also allows poisonous wastes, which the liver has removed from the body, to be eliminated through the intestines.

Many people fail to have free, unobstructed flow of bile from the liver and gall bladder. Eating processed food, eating unprocessed food which is mineral-deficient, and experiencing lack of regular exercise, stress, and worry during meals, all combine to alter the chemistry of bile. Consequently, formation of solid particles forming from bile is a common occurrence. These solid particles remain in the gall bladder, or the base of the liver, for many years. They become progressively harder, often congealing into "gallstones." Long before this occurs, however, metabolic problems are underway. When a significant number of solid bile particles accumulate, the free flow of the gall bladder's contents is diminished, causing progressive stagnation and congestion of the liver.

The importance of cleansing the debris from the liver and gall bladder, thus keeping the bile free-flowing, is often emphasized by metabolic doctors. This can be effectively accomplished by doing the liver-gall bladder flush, which is described in this chapter's addendum. The liver-gall bladder flush is said to be a highly effective detoxification measure, one that stimulates the liver's function tremendously.

Keeping this natural flow of toxins moving through the liver is as essential for cancer resistance as it is for general health. Jesse Greenstein wrote in *Biochemistry of Cancer,* "There seems to be little doubt that hepatic (liver) insufficiency is a concomitant phenomenon with cancer. . . ."[10]

Dr. Max Gerson, a pioneer in the development of metabolic therapy for cancer, believed that the liver was the body's most important organ in defeating developed malignancy. He also believed that almost all cancers were allowed to develop because of poor function of the liver. "During the first stage—development and appearance of the disease (cancer)—the liver dysfunction is undetectable," he wrote in *A Cancer Therapy*.[11] "During the second stage—tumor growth and some metastases in glands—one finds the liver mostly hypertrophic (enlarged), and, as we see in some cases, there is also hypertrophy or edema of other organs. In the third stage we see an almost entire autonomy of the cancer, with rapid poisoning, destruction and later dissolution of the organs, including the liver, which can no longer maintain its substance and functions."[12]

Among the stresses on the liver, Greenstein said, is "the production by the tumor of a circulating toxin which accelerates the catabolism (breakdown) of the body tissues," including those in the liver.[13]

Dr. Gerson stated that, "Detoxification is abolutely necessary, and the greatest therapeutical help for the liver. Healing is limited or even impossible in cases where the liver is no longer able to . . . maintain its vital service. . . ."[14]

Dr. Gerson believed in stimulating liver function in cancer patients with, among other procedures, the coffee enema. Metabolic doctors associated with Dr. Kelley also are avid believers in the efficacy of coffee enemas. They recommend that cancer patients do a coffee enema once or twice daily, throughout their therapy. The procedure, described in detail in the chapter addendum, is essentially a 15 to 30 minute retention enema that uses approximately one quart of lukewarm, organic, unsprayed coffee. Its mechanism of action is the entrance of caffeine directly into the liver, via the portal vein, which connects the colon and liver. This influx of caffeine stimulates the liver to discharge large volumes of toxic waste into the bile, so that these toxins can be eliminated from the system. Little of the caffeine enters the general system, causing very infrequent feelings of overstimulation in most people. Patients almost universally report a rapid increase in feelings of energy and improved emotional outlook after a coffee enema, not because of a caffeine "high," but because of elimination of toxins from the bloodstream, the cells and the liver itself. Healthy people often report an improved state of feeling after a coffee enema, and the benefits for cancer patients derived from this easily-applied procedure are frequently dramatic. The procedure dispels nausea, feelings of irritability, lethargy, lack of appetite and sometimes even severe pain. The procedure appears to soothe and calm the nervous system. It is said that in World War I the Germans administered coffee enemas to painfully wounded soldiers when there was no morphine.

"In the beginning of treatment," wrote Dr. Gerson, "some patients vomit a great amount of bile and suffer a kind of toxic diarrhea." When they were given coffee enemas, however, he said, "these violent reactions no longer occurred."[15] Dr. Gerson said that "enemas also help against spasms, precordial pain, and difficulties resulting from the sudden withdrawal of all intoxicating agents. . . . Difficult as this may be to believe, experience has proved that frequent enemas completely eliminate the need for sedation."[16]

Robert Bradford writes in *Now That You Have Cancer,* "The coffee enema is an excellent way to provide quick, effective detoxification."

Another advantage of the procedure is that it also stimulates the pancreas, creating greater insulin output, which makes the body's cell walls more permeable, and also creates greater enzyme output.

Most immunotherapeutic and metabolic therapists employ coffee enemas. The procedure has been endorsed by Dr. Bernard Jensen, Dr. Ernesto Contreras, Dr. John Richardson, Dr. Richard Passwater and a great many others.

It should be mentioned that recent claims were made that coffee enemas were the cause of death of two persons in the Seattle area, presumably because the enemas somehow imbalanced the biochemistry of those people. It is, the author feels, probably less than coincidental that the two people who died were both terminally ill cancer patients. Having discussed this procedure with a great many of the metabolic physicians in America who regularly employ it, and having heard of virtually no negative reactions to coffee enemas, it seems clear to the author that reports of the supposed "dangers" of coffee enemas are essentially ill-founded.

Patients sometimes resist the idea of coffee enemas. Many people, it seems, have an emotional aversion to discussing, or trying to regulate, functions related to their bowel area. Even Dr. Passwater admits that the idea of coffee enemas "sounded strange to me at one time."[17] There is also probably some resistance to the procedure because it makes therapeutic use of coffee, which is generally thought of as a harmful stimulant. There is, furthermore, a fear amongst patients that they will become "addicted" to enemas, and become unable to have regular bowel movements (the fear is totally unfounded; coffee enemas actually strengthen peristaltic lower bowel function).

In almost all people who try the procedure, these negative feelings, according to metabolic doctors, are overcome after the first coffee enema. The procedure is simply so refreshing and energizing that patients feel they can't afford to hang onto their prejudices and misconceptions about coffee enemas. The coffee enema is considered as important as any other single facet of a metabolic program—it's considered as important as, for example, vitamin C, or a low protein diet, or a positive outlook. It is considered truly a powerful weapon for stimulating the liver, and as Luanne Rona, M.D., says, "The word liver means life, and there probably isn't another word that could describe it better."[18]

For a description of the coffee enema procedure, see the chapter addendum.

Cleaning the Kidneys and Skin

The kidneys and skin are two other important organs of elimination. We sometimes don't think of the skin as an eliminative organ, but it has earned a nickname in medical circles as "the third kidney."

The kidneys are vital organs of detoxification. They filter approximately 4,000 quarts of blood daily. Metabolic wastes, largely in the form of urea, are eliminated in the urine. Discharge of urea also helps maintain the body's acid/alkaline balance. Many drugs are eliminated through the kidneys, including pharmaceutical analgesics and non-prescription analgesics, such as aspirin.

The kidneys can respond to toxic overload with nephritis, a kidney disease, or can form kidney stones, which are composed of oxalic acid and calcium. Kidney failure is difficult to notice in its early stages, and thus difficult to deter. The kidneys are a very regenerative organ, though, and can be helped to heal with dietary support and flushing with clean liquids. Drs. Edwin Prien and Stanley Gershoff reported to health science writer and editor Mark Bricklin that they were able to successfully dissolve kidney debris, including crystallized stones, with a simple nutritional formula.[19]

Large volumes of waste products exit the body via the kidneys, and they can become overloaded, according to metabolic doctors, during rapid elimination of toxins during recovery from cancer. Severe overloading of the kidneys can cause them to reject toxins, sending harmful substances back into the bloodstream. Toxic build-up in the kidneys can also result in infection or gradual deterioration, both of which can contribute to a downward spiral of systemic toxicity. Metabolic doctors say that it is important that the cancer patient keep the kidneys free of toxic build-up, in order to maintain the outward flow of toxins through urinary expulsion.

To achieve this, it is be helpful to use mild herbal diuretics, and to flush the kidneys by consuming relatively large amounts of pure juice and water, and to avoid use of excessive salt, which causes fluid retention. Avoiding impure water is considered especially important in the flushing procedure, since even small amounts of copper, cadmium and lead, frequently present in city water supplies, can toxify the kidneys, then be absorbed into the system. For details on kidney cleansing techniques, see the chapter addendum.

The skin, which excretes toxins through perspiration, has eliminative functions similar to those of the kidneys, and is prone to similar problems. A common occurrence for cancer patients who begin to expel toxins, say metabolic doctors, is to break out in skin blemishes. This is a positive healing crisis, they say, since it signifies expulsion of toxic agents through the epidermal layer. Sometimes these eruptions are accompanied by an unpleasant odor emanating from the skin, which is further evidence, say the doctors, of the voiding of poisons and necrotic cellular material through the skin.

It is considered important to keep the skin's pores as open as possible, because this encourages further elimination from the internal cells. The skin's eliminative functions are stimulated with various forms of bathing; controlled sweating with saunas, hot baths, sunbathing and steam baths; application of compresses, clays and "wet packs"; and dry skin brushing. These procedures are all as pleasant and relaxing as they are health propitiating.

Keeping the surface of the skin clean is also important, since some bacteria, when put in direct contact with other bacteria, exchange genetic material and form newer, more virulent strains. Dr. Stanley Falkow of the University of Washington calls these 'jumping genes.'"[20]

"The skin," says Dian Buchman, in *Water Therapy,* "is the largest organ for elimination, and simple emersion in a long, hot bath or a sauna or steamroom can stimulate excretion of toxins from the body through the skin. The inducing of perspiration is useful in treating acute diseases and many chronic health problems."[21]

"The skin," says Luanne Rona, M.D., "has been grossly overlooked in its importance in eliminating body waste material. Under chemical analysis, the composition (of perspiration) shows a high content of uric acid (a metabolic waste product), which is also a component of urine.

"When the pores of the skin become choked and filled with debris and dead cells, the powerful waste eliminating ability of the skin is impaired. The consequence is that more work is required by the kidneys and liver. In a body with a heavy skin layer, approximately a pound of waste matter can be expelled through it daily. From the Finnish saunas to the ancient Roman Baths, one can see the early understanding of the healing powers of sweating. . . ."[22]

For skin-stimulating procedures, see the chapter addendum.

Detoxifying the Colon and Lungs

The colon, or large intestine, is under constant toxic stress, since it is responsible for evacuating fecal matter from the body. People eating a common American diet, extremely high in refined carbohydrates and fats, are placing an almost insurmountable burden upon their colons. It is no wonder that colon cancer is the most common form of cancer in men/women combined, and that almost the entire population suffers, to some degree, from diverticulosis (pockets protruding from the colon wall).

The significance of detoxifying the colon for a cancer patient, say metabolic doctors, is in the general benefit his or her entire system will derive. If the patient has colon cancer, of course, more specific benefits are said to be accrued.

The colon wall, from years of eating refined, difficult to digest foods, becomes encrusted, in almost all persons living in a technological society, with a coating of largely impermeable, often hardened mucous and waste material. This coating attracts further build-up of waste, traps toxins within the system, and blocks absorption of minerals, which the body receives through colonic absorption.[23] Professor Arnold Ehret writes in the *Mucusless Diet Healing System* that autopsies have revealed that "from 60 to 70 per cent of the colons examined have foreign matters, such as . . . decades-old feces" stored in them. "The average, so-called 'healthy' man of today," writes Ehret, "carries continually with him, since childhood, several pounds of never-eliminated feces."[24]

Colonic therapist Barbara Poe, R.N., concurs with the grim assessment of Professor Ehret. "Most people simply do not eliminate all of the waste that their body processes. They retain parts of it indefinitely. This is, of course, detrimental to their general health, since substances from a toxic colon are reabsorbed into the bloodstream."[25] Poe says that a significant number of the patients who consult her are cancer patients, and that virtually all of them benefit from colonic irrigation.

Cancer patient Eydie Mae describes the colonic irrigation procedure: "The colonic rectal speculum (the inserting tube) is a single tube that is inserted into the rectum, which has two rubber tubes extending from it. One tube is attached to the incoming water supply and the other is attached to the outflow of the bowel content, so that there is a constant inflow and outflow through the mechanism. The water is warmed to body temperature or slightly warmer. The pressure of the inflow and outflow is also controlled. The water irrigates the bowel, and the waste material and toxins are carried out while the patient is very comfortably lying down. It is not unpleasant at all."[26] Most metabolic doctors recommend that seriously ill people have a colonic about once a week or more often if desired.

The coffee enema is also a very efficient means of cleaning

the lower bowel of accumulated toxins. The coffee dissolves old, encrusted wastes. Other forms of enemas, with wheatgrass, flaxseed, distilled water, a yogurt or buttermilk solution, or apple cider vinegar are recommended by Dr. Bernard Jensen and others as effective lower bowel detoxifiers.[27]

Fasting can be very helpful, especially when combined with colonic irrigations or coffee enemas. Metabolic doctors recommend that cancer patients do not fast without engaging in other simultaneous detoxification measures, because elimination must keep pace with the accelerated cell-turnover that is likely to accompany a fast. Dr. Jack Goldstein writes of cancer patients, in *Triumph Over Disease by Fasting,* that fasting can "relieve the patient's pain. . . ."[28] Cancer therapist George Crile, M.D., has written that he believes that, in fasting, "one of the great hopes for the future lies. It is possible that ultimately cancer will be controlled not by attacking the cancer, but by starving it or altering the environment in which it lives."[29] For instructions on fasts, see the chapter addendum.

The lungs represent the final organ of elimination, and probably the most overlooked. The lungs, however, in their expulsion of carbon dioxide, also expel many other gaseous wastes and solid mucous-carried wastes. Metabolic doctors say that it is not unusual for a cancer patient, once his or her healing process begins, to have bad breath during healing crises, especially if detoxification procedures are not adequately employed.

"The lung structure" says Dr. Bernard Jensen, "is a vital one because it is a great catch-point for catarrh, phlegm and mucous, which settle in the chest as part of the eliminative process. . . . Accumulated toxins in the bowel are thrown back into the body, absorbed by the blood, and finally go to the lung structure. This is where we have large amounts thrown off in a hurry. I have seen some people throw off teaspoons of catarrh through the bronchial tubes. This is something we do not try to stop. We try to bring about more of it. . . ."[30]

Breathing exercises are almost always of benefit to people who are ill, say metabolic doctors, including those who have cancer. Breathing exercises stimulate optimum function of the lungs. When the alveolar sacs and ducts are expanded, and blood is forced into the tissues, and rapid air exchange is brought about, the eliminative function of the lungs is accelerated. "Aerobic" exercises, which stimulate deep breathing, have been shown to increase conversion of oxygen in the body by up to 50 per cent.[31] See the chapter addendum for specific breathing exercises.

Combined Detoxification

It is considered important to engage simultaneously in detoxification of all the organs of elimination, since they are all so obviously related. Fasts, purges, enemas, liver flushes, saunas, baths and exercise are thought to synergistically combine to lessen the toxic burden on the body. As one becomes increasingly less toxic, and increasingly cancer-free, life will be immeasurably more enjoyable.

Special Information: "Detoxification"

Detoxification Procedures

Please note: the following procedures were described to the author by physicians who regularly employ these procedures as part of a complex health-building metabolic program. Patients should consult a physician before engaging in any of these procedures. The author makes no therapeutic claims for any of these procedures.

The Liver-Gall Bladder Flush

The four basic elements in this procedure are:

1. Apple juice (high in malic acid) or orthophosphoric acid, which act as solvents in the bile to weaken adhesions between solid globules.

2. Epsom Salt (magnesium sulfate), taken by mouth and enema, which allows magnesium to be absorbed into the bloodstream, relaxing smooth muscles. Large solid particles which otherwise might create spasms are allowed to pass through a relaxed bile duct, if Epsom Salt is used.

3. Olive oil or other unrefined oil, which stimulates the gall bladder and bile duct to contract powerfully, thus expelling solid particles kept in storage for years.

4. Coffee enemas, which consist of a coffee solution retained in the colon. They activate the liver to secrete its waste into the bile, enhancing bile flow and further relaxing the bile duct muscle.

One of the most important procedures for persons over ten years of age is the liver-gall bladder flush. If one is above ten years of age and his or her physician gives approval, he or she should do this the first week of a metabolic program, and should, with the physician's approval, repeat it every two months. The steps in doing this are as follows:

1. For five days prior to the "flush," consume as much apple juice or cider as the appetite permits, in addition to regular meals. Add a total of 90 drops of a phosphorus solution to the apple juice or cider each day. The juice and phosphorus will soften the gall bladder debris and facilitate egress. Nutritional supplements should also be taken during this time. The best juice would be freshly juiced, from organic apples, and secondly, apple juice or cider (unsweetened and preferably organic if possible) purchased from the health food or grocery store. A person should read the labels carefully and obtain a juice that has no sugar or additives.

If one is severely hypoglycemic, is diabetic, or has difficulty tolerating the juice or cider, take 30 drops of a phosphorus solution with each meal (90 drops daily) in distilled water or some type of juice other than apple. Due to the high acidity, it is wise to brush one's teeth or rinse the mouth with Milk of Magnesia after taking the orthophosphoric acid.

2. At noon on the sixth day, one should eat a normal lunch and take the supplements scheduled for that time.

3. Two hours after lunch, two tablespoons of Epsom Salt should be taken, dissolved in one to three ounces of mineral water or distilled water. The taste may be objectionable. If so, the mixture can be followed by a little citrus juice, if desired (freshly squeezed if possible).

4. Four hours after lunch, one should take a one-quart coffee enema with one-fourth cup of Epsom Salt dissolved in it. This should be retained for 15 minutes and then expelled. The coffee should be made as strong as one can tolerate, but no stronger than four tablespoons of ground coffee per quart of water.

5. Five hours after lunch, take one tablespoon of Epsom Salt, dissolved as the previous dose.

6. Six or seven hours after lunch, one may fast if desired. However, it is preferable to have a fresh fruit salad, using as many fresh fruits in season as possible. Use heavy whipping cream as dressing on the salad, whipped with a little honey if desired. One can eat as much as desired of the whipped cream-covered salad. If fresh fruit is unavailable, frozen berries, such as strawberries, blueberries, boysenberries, blackberries, raspberries, etc., can be used. These should also be covered with

whipped cream. Take citrus fruit or juice after the cream and fruit meal, if desired. For hypoglycemics, the cream will balance the fruit. However, hypoglycemics should adjust the amount of salad to their individual tolerance.

7. At bedtime, there can be one of three choices:

a. Take one-half cup of unrefined olive or other oil followed by a small glass of orange, grapefruit, or lemon juice. (All juice should be freshly squeezed.)

b. Take one-half cup of unrefined olive or other oil blended with one-half cup of orange, grapefruit, or diluted lemon juice.

c. Take two tablespoons of unrefined olive or other oil followed by two tablespoons of citrus juice every 15 minutes until eight ounces of it has been consumed. (This choice is preferable for those who are unusually weak or who have had gall bladder problems in the past.)

If one should vomit during the consumption of the oil and juice, the procedure should be continued until it is finished. It is not necessary to make up for the amount that was vomited. Nausea felt during this process indicates stimulation of the gall bladder and/or liver.

8. Immediately upon finishing the oil and juice (or while taking it), one should go to bed and lie on the right side with the right knee drawn up toward the chin for 20 minutes before going to sleep. This encourages the oil to drain from the stomach, helping contents of the gall bladder and/or liver to move into the small intestine.

9. If one feels quite ill during the night, another strong coffee enema with the Epsom Salt may be taken.

10. If there is a strong feeling of nausea the following morning, one should try to remain in bed until it subsides somewhat. Vomiting should not be forced.

11. Upon arising, one must take another strong coffee enema with Epsom Salt in it or, one hour before breakfast, take one tablespoon of Epsom Salt dissolved in one to three ounces of mineral water or distilled water.

12. If one continues to feel nauseous or very sore in the upper abdomen even after the enema, a light diet of sprouts, fruit (raw or steamed), yogurt or kefir, and freshly extracted vegetable juices (especially with beet greens in them) should be

maintained for several days until one feels better. Then gradually resume the normal diet. If one finds that the supplements cause discomfort immediately after the flush, they may be omitted for three days.

One should not be frightened by the above references to nausea, vomiting, soreness of the abdomen, etc. Chances are that the symptoms won't be severe enough to cause vomiting or soreness of the abdomen; this happens only very rarely. Many people complete this procedure with minimal discomfort, and nearly everyone feels much better after completing it. Flushing of the liver and gall bladder stimulates and cleans these organs extremely efficiently.

Often, persons suffering from gallstones, lack of appetite, biliousness, backaches, nausea, and a host of other complaints for years will find gallstone-type objects in the stool the day following the flush. These objects are light to dark green in color, very irregular in shape, gelatinous in texture, and of sizes varying from "grape seeds" to "cherries." If there seems to be a large number of these objects in the stool, the flush should be repeated in two weeks.

Exercises for the Colon

Exercise of all kinds aids colon function; whatever type is most enjoyable should be engaged in regularly. One exercise specifically beneficial for the colon is the abdominal lift. To do this, bend down slightly, placing both hands on the knees. All the breath should be exhaled forcefully through the mouth. Remain at full exhalation and pull the stomach muscles in, relax, and pull in again, visualizing bringing the navel back to the spine. This should be done 10 to 15 times, then the abdominal muscles should be relaxed and normal breathing should be resumed. When breathing is comfortable, the semicrouched position should be resumed, all the breath exhaled, and the exercise repeated.

It is helpful to try a rolling motion when pulling in the abdomen, first bringing in the lower part and rolling upward toward the ribs. The abdominal lifts should be done in three or four sets on arising, after the coffee enema (often this helps in expelling the last portions of it), and before meals—never on a full stomach. They are particularly good for those with the common situation of prolapse (sagging) of the transverse colon. The abdominal muscles used in the exercise gently massage and lift the transverse colon, and tone all the organs of the digestive tract.

There is another simple maneuver that can be done regularly, before and after the daily enema, and before meals, to prevent malfunctioning of the "ileocecal valve," a sphincter muscle between the ileum (last part of the small intestine) and the cecum (first part of the ascending colon), located just above the appendix. This valve is designed to be a one-way valve that lets digested food contents move from the small intestine to the colon, where the food is further broken down and acted upon by bacteria in the colon. Sudden addition of fiber to the diet, mechanical stress from the enema, and many complex neurological factors can cause the ileocecal valve to open, which allows reverse flow of waste material and bacteria into the small intestine. There it is absorbed, producing sudden headache, nausea, back, chest, or shoulder pain, and other symptoms. This is easily prevented by the following: Place the right hand over the appendix (if the little finger is placed just on the protruding hip bone, the second, third and fourth fingers will be well positioned). While breathing in, press in and gently stretch the skin and underlying tissue toward the left shoulder with the first three fingers. The breath should be exhaled and released seven to eight times. The ileocecal valve can also be closed by placing a pint sized cannister of cold water (kept in the refrigerator for this purpose) over the ileocecal valve area.

An important factor in colon function is proper acid/alkaline balance. The colon should be slightly acidic. If it becomes alkaline, the gas forming organisms become active and a large amount of foul-smelling gas is produced.

Foods which help maintain an acid condition in the colon are all the lactic acid and fermented foods, such as acidophilus yogurt, lactobacillus bifidus, sauerkraut and pickles.

Purging

The stored toxins and metabolic wastes which are released on a daily basis as a metabolic program is followed are very acid-forming. If they accumulate, they inhibit the efficiency of important enzymes in the blood, which are favored by a slightly alkaline medium. To give the body, and especially the organs of digestion and elimination, a rest, and to cleanse it of these acid wastes, it is recommended that a one-day purge, followed by one day of fasting, be done at least every other month (alternating with the liver-gall bladder flush).

Immediately upon rising, one should take a coffee enema. One-half hour after the coffee enema is expelled, one should take one tablespoon of Epsom Salt, dissolved in two to four ounces of distilled water. In 30 minutes, this should be repeated. In another 30 minutes, it should be repeated once again, making three doses in all.

After at least two hours, and as one becomes hungry, one may take an alkalizing punch—one glass or more every hour, or as desired. Make the punch by putting the juice of six fresh lemons, 12 oranges, and six grapefruit in a gallon glass jar and filling the rest of the jar with distilled water. No food or supplements are eaten during a day of purging, except for an orange or grapefruit in the evening.

The purge should be repeated on the following day, and the entire two-day process repeated once every two months. (In case of extreme weakness, take the purge only one day each time.)

During the purge, the body may undergo some rather uncomfortable sensations such as nausea, headaches, cramps and dizziness. These are a result of the cleansing. Poisons that have accumulated for years are suddenly excreted, and this is a shock to the system. These sensations are temporary and will disappear when the toxins are finally removed from the body. Severe hypoglycemics should consult a metabolic physician before this procedure.

Fasting

After the purge, a fast must be started. It should also last for two days, unless one is too weak, in which case one day of fasting is sufficient, until one's strength is built up. A fast gives one's body a rest and an opportunity to cleanse itself of much waste on the individual cell level. As in the purge, some discomfort may be experienced after the fast or during it. Each day of the fast, one quart of fresh carrot juice should be taken, along with all the distilled water desired. Grape, cherry or apple juice may be taken in place of carrot juice, if the carrot juice cannot be adequately digested. Any of these juices may be diluted with equal parts of distilled water, or enough water to suit one's taste.

Unless sufficient fluids are taken, toxins become concentrated and are not eliminated sufficiently. The coffee enema should be taken once or twice during the day of fasting.

Potato peel broth (high in potassium) is often helpful on a day of fasting, and may be taken as desired.

The outer one-fourth inch of three medium-sized, organically grown potatoes should be peeled, placed in a stainless steel pan, covered with a quart of distilled water, and simmered for 20 minutes.

This may be seasoned as one pleases, preferably with Dr. Bronner's Balanced Mineral Salt (obtainable at health food stores), which is made from seaweed and is also high in potassium.

No other food or supplements should be taken on a day of fasting.

For severe hypoglycemics, the fast will have to be modified by taking six to ten tablets of a high-quality protein tablet every two hours. Soy protein tablets or powders are not acceptable.

For three days following the fast, it is often helpful to take one or two tablespoons of apple cider vinegar in four to six ounces of distilled water with the second and third meals. If this causes burning or discomfort, it should be either discontinued or diluted with more water. After taking the vinegar, the mouth should be rinsed well with Milk of Magnesia to neutralize excess acidity.

Lactic acid yeast is very helpful in restoring intestinal flora after the fast. It also helps reduce the excess gas that many people will experience. Take two tablets with each meal, indefinitely, or for as long as experiencing excessive gas. This lactic acid yeast is entirely different from brewer's or other types of yeast. Substitutions with any other than this particular product will not be useful.

Enemas and Colonic Irrigations

A high enema, using coffee, should be taken every day. The coffee enema is very stimulating to the liver and is the greatest aid in elimination of the liver's toxic wastes.

If colonic irrigations are available, they should be taken once a week for the first three months in addition to the coffee enemas, and occasionally after that, depending upon the severity of the cancer. The advice of the person giving the colonic irrigations should be followed.

It is best to arise early enough each morning to allow time to take the enema in a relaxed, unhurried state. Steps for proper procedure are:

1. Upon rising, make a pot of coffee. The coffee must be regular, non-instant, non-decaffeinated coffee. It must be prepared in enamelware, Corning Ware, glass or stainless steel, or by use of the tricolator filter method. Aluminum or Teflon should not be used at any time. Some metabolic physicians have found that coffee which is unboiled or prepared via the "drip method" is preferable. Use two to four tablespoons of ground coffee to one quart of distilled water. Any water that enters the body should be distilled.

If a coffee enema makes a person jittery, shaky, nervous, nauseated, or lightheaded, the solution is too strong. The amount of coffee can be adjusted from one teaspoon to four tablespoons per quart of distilled water as the tolerance level permits.

Some people, children especially, can retain only a pint of enema solution at a time. If this is the case, one must take two enemas each time, one right after the other, and hold each for 15 minutes.

If one has a limited time schedule in the mornings, the coffee may be made the night before and warmed to body temperature the next morning.

2. While the coffee is cooling to body or room temperature, do some form of mild exercise such as walking briskly, or even light jogging if one is strong and energetic enough. If one is extremely debilitated and weak, this step, will, of course, need to be omitted until strength returns.

3. Attempt a normal bowel movement. The enema is much

more effective if the colon has been evacuated. One should not become disturbed, however, if there are no regular bowel movements, or very few, during this program. In many cases, not enough bulk collects to instigate a normal bowel movement. When no normal bowel movements are forthcoming, the enema cleans the colon adequately.

Bulk formers, such as Metamucil (obtainable at drug stores), or two tablespoons of miller's bran (obtainable at health food stores), taken with each meal are quite helpful in forming stools. Occasionally, when cancer is in the abdomen, the intestinal tract will become obstructed. Usually, under these circumstances, no food or feces will come through. After a few days the patient becomes extremely nauseated and starts vomiting. He or she will be very sick and will normally run a high temperature. This should be watched quite carefully, for in such cases immediate emergency measures are necessary.

One should never allow himself or herself to become extremely toxic, in order to be able to distinguish between a healing toxic reaction and an intestinal obstruction. As soon as nausea or vomiting develops and no food is passing through, all supplements and food should be stopped for five days. Water and juice may be taken during this time. If there is no vomiting, food is passing through, and the temperature remains below 100 degrees, the diet and normal routine may be resumed, as one may assume there is no obstruction. If, during the five days off the supplements with no solid food intake, one begins to vomit and has abdominal pain with high temperature, a physician should be consulted to check for intestinal obstruction.

4. After the normal bowel movement, or before taking the coffee retention enema, most people find that taking an enema with warm distilled water is very helpful. This procedure begins the cleansing of the colon, removing large particles of residue and most of the gas. When it is completed, the coffee retention enema may be taken. The warm water enema is optional and does not need to be taken if the coffee enema can be retained for the desired period.

5. When the coffee has cooled to body or room temperature, pour it into an enema or douche bag. The enema tip on the end of the hose is not adequate to give a "high enema." A 30-inch colon tube should be used on the plastic enema nozzle.

This colon tube can be purchased from a drug store or hospital supply outlet, or from Answer Pharmacy.

A. The colon tube should be lubricated with natural creamery butter, Vitamin E cream, or other lubricant that doesn't contain additives or chemicals.

B. Allow the coffee to flow to the end of the colon tube, thus eliminating any air in the tube.

C. Insert the tube 18 to 30 inches into the rectum, if possible. This should be done slowly, in a rotating motion that helps to keep the tube from kinking up inside the colon.

D. There are several positions that can be used while inserting the colon tube. Squatting is one. There is also the knee-chest method, with chest and knees on the floor and buttocks in the highest position possible. Most people, however, find it easiest to lie on the left side until the solution is out of the bag. The enema should never be taken while sitting on the toilet or standing.

E. Some people's colons have turns or obstructions that may prevent the tube from being inserted even 18 inches. Often, if a little bit of the solution is allowed to flow into the colon as the tube is being inserted, one can comfortably get past these obstructions.

F. If an obstruction bends the tube too much and stops the flow of liquid, then the tube can be inserted only as far as it will go, still allowing the liquid to flow freely.

G. Sometimes, if one hits an obstruction that stops the flow of liquid completely, the tube can be pulled out slowly just to the point where the solution flows again. Frequently, the tube can be pushed back in, past the turn that previously stopped the liquid.

H. Because of the shapes and formations of some people's colons, or, of course, if a child is being given the enema, it will be possible to insert the tube only a few inches. Occasionally, this is a permanent situation. Often, however, as the colon is cleansed and healed, the tube can eventually be inserted further.

I. The tube should never be forced when discomfort occurs.

J. The enema or douche bag should not be over 18 inches higher than the rectum. If it is placed too high, the coffee runs into the colon too fast and under too much pressure, causing discomfort.

K. After the flow of the solution is completed, one may remove the colon tube, although it isn't necessary to do so. Regardless of the position used up to this point, one now should lie on the left side for at least five minutes, then on the back for another five minutes, then on the right side for at least five minutes.

L. Those who have excessive gas may leave the tube in the colon with the hose clamp open. This allows the gas to escape through the enema apparatus. Frequently, the coffee will go in and out of the enema bag until the gas is relieved.

M. After the enema is retained for 15 minutes or longer, it may be expelled. Massage of the abdominal area is sometimes helpful for full expulsion.

Cleaning the Kidneys

The kidneys should be flushed each day with liberal quantities of fluid, either distilled water or fresh fruit and vegetable juices (preferably organic). Parsley tea is excellent for strengthening the kidneys. Ordinary commercial teas and coffee should be avoided by those with kidney problems. Herbal teas are acceptable.

For those who tend to retain fluid, watermelon is an excellent diuretic. If the melon is organically grown, the rind should be juiced and sipped first thing in the morning and then the red fleshy part of the fruit may be eaten. Two mornings a week, one may take the juice of a whole lemon in warm distilled water as a diuretic (citrus should not be used more than two days a week, as it tends to upset the calcium-phosphorus metabolism if used more frequently). Shavegrass or horsetail tea are good diuretics and also good for the skin and hair. An excellent diuretic salad may be made by combining cabbage and onions—finely sliced—with crushed raw garlic; parsley, and herbs like sage, cumin, and juniper berries, if available. Cover this mixture with very hot distilled water and place a lid over it for ten minutes. Drain the mixture (the liquid is good to save for soup bases, grains, etc.) and squeeze a lemon over it. It can be eaten as is or refrigerated first. It can also be mixed with other salads.

In extreme fluid retention, one's physician may prescribe a diuretic drug, which is permissible, and the doctor will normally increase the intake of potassium to compensate for its loss on account of the drug.

Cleaning the Lungs

If there is excessive accumulation of mucus in the nostrils and/or bronchial system, this inhibits the detoxification functions of the lungs. Mucus-forming foods should be avoided if mucus is a problem. These are principally dairy products, with the exception of butter and cream, and baked flour products. Anti-mucus foods, such as raw onions and garlic, cayenne pepper, freshly ground black pepper, fresh ginger, and horseradish should be eaten liberally.

Irrigating the Nostrils

Salt water irrigation of the nostrils is very helpful in dispelling nasal mucus and sinus congestion. If one cannot breathe through the nose, one is bypassing a crucial filtering mechanism which warms and humidifies the air and which removes large amounts of toxic particulants and dust before this air reaches the back of one's throat. Mouth-breathing places incalculable stress on the lungs, nearly equivalent to that of cigarette smoking, if one lives in urban pollution.

To irrigate the nostrils, dissolve one teaspoon of sea salt in 16 ounces of warm water, in a bowl of appropriate size. While bending forward, block one nostril and place the other below the water surface in the bowl. The water should be gently drawn up the nostril until one can taste the salty mixture trickling to the back of the throat, then it should be blown out. This should be repeated with the other nostril and alternated several times.

Breathing Exercises

Breathing exercises should follow the cleansing of the nostrils. If done on a regular basis, these yield tremendous benefits. They increase the body's supply of oxygen (which is the basic currency for repair and for burning up toxins), increase the removal of waste products and stagnant air from portions of the lungs otherwise unused, and exercise the diaphragm—which serves as a pump for the flow of oxygen and energy. Deep breathing Exercise No. 1 yields a multitude of benefits through maximum use of lung capacity. Rapid breathing Exercise No. 2 is an energizing exercise which promotes flow of energy into the lungs and digestive organs. It should be done before meals, after being in a stuffy room, or whenever extra energy is desired.

Alternate-nostril breathing Exercise No. 3 has a calming effect on the nervous system. It can be used effectively to overcome anxiety states and insomnia, and sometimes to relieve headaches.

Any sitting posture may be used for performing the breathing exercises. It is important to keep the spine straight and chest wall spread to not impede the body's natural tendency to expand upon inhalation. The body should be kept straight and steady, but relaxed, with the hands on the knees or in the lap (unless otherwise indicated).

Because one is dealing with such delicate organs as the lungs, heart and nerve centers, one should take great care not to strain any part of the system by overdoing this practice.

Deep Breathing Exercise No. 1

Sit comfortably with the spine erect but relaxed. Inhale and exhale through the nose slowly. As one inhales, the stomach should be expanded first and then the chest wall, to allow in the maximum amount of air. One may raise the collarbones also. The abdominal muscles will automatically contract a little as the chest becomes full. Then, without holding the breath, one should exhale slowly. The collarbones should be dropped first; then the chest should be contracted; and lastly, the stomach should be contracted—one action flowing into the other. In both inhalation and exhalation, the breath should be one continuous flow. The cycle should be repeated slowly and steadily. This method fills the lungs to capacity and empties them thoroughly.

One may imagine one's breath to be like an elevator. Every inhalation begins from the ground floor (stomach) and goes through the second floor (rib cage) and finally to the third floor (upper chest), and every exhalation goes back down from the top floor to the middle floor, to the ground floor. One may feel that one's body is a balloon being filled up as one inhales (expands), and when one exhales, the air leaves the balloon.

Rapid Breathing Exercise No. 2

This technique utilizes just one part of the body, as differentiated from the deep breathing that uses the entire thorax. Here we use just an inhalation into the stomach, letting it expand outward, and a quick and forceful exhalation, pulling the stomach in and forcing the air up and out through the nose to produce a sneezelike sound. Alternation of exhalation and inhalation should continue in a rapid fashion, creating a movement like that of bellows. One should begin with a few inhalations and exhalations per group, gradually increasing the number according to one's capacity. One to three groups should be done in any sitting, with rest in between groups, and with a deep inhalation and a slow exhalation at the end of each group.

It is helpful in the beginning of this practice to have one hand resting on the stomach to feel the in-and-out bellows-like movement. When comfortable with the exercise, it is more helpful to have hands on knees, to help keep the posture steady. There is a tendency to move the shoulders up and down, as well as the chest, but the only movement should be in the abdomen. If any dizziness results from this practice, one should stop and take a slow deep breath and then continue more slowly after a rest. This exercise is very cleansing for the body and eliminates impurities from the lungs and nasal passages, as well as building a gentle heat which helps burn and eliminate toxins throughout the body.

Alternate-Nostril Breathing Exercise No. 3

This is similar to the deep breathing, with the single addition of alternating nostrils as one breathes, inhaling through one at a time, by closing the other off with fingers. A helpful aid is to form a fist of the right hand and have only the last two fingers and thumb extended, leaving the other fingers tucked into the base of the thumb. The thumb should then be brought up to the right nostril, closing it off to permit exhaling through the left nostril. Then, after the exhalation, without any sudden jerk, one should begin slowly inhaling through the same left nostril—taking a slow, steady, deep breath. Now one should change nostrils by closing the left nostril with the last two fingers and releasing the thumb. Exhalation should be started slowly and steadily. Now again, one should inhale and then switch nostrils, exhale, inhale, and switch, going through five to ten cycles. One can count as one breathes, letting exhalation be twice as long as inhalation. This exercise aids digestion and seems to calm and balance the nervous system.

Cleaning the Skin

To open the pores and remove dead skin, skin brushing before a shower and vigorous use of a loofah sponge in the shower are recommended. A good quality vegetable-bristle skin brush should be purchased from the health food store or pharmacy. One should brush up the front of the body and down the back, over all exposed skin surfaces, until a warm glow is felt. Then one should take a warm shower and rub briskly with a loofah sponge (available in most health food stores) to remove the layers of dead skin loosened by the brushing.

Castile or other pure soap should be used in bathing, but in minimal amount, since heavy soaking will wash off all the valuable skin oils and can cause the skin to overproduce oil in order to compensate. The hair should be shampooed frequently with a non-chemical soap or shampoo, which can be found in health food stores.

At the end of a shower, one should turn the water to cool, then to warm. As one becomes accustomed to the temperature change, one may go from hot to cold and back several times. This exercises the tiny muscles in the skin which control dilation and contraction of the pores. As they become stronger, they can respond better to the physiological demands of the body.

After the shower, one can sit in a tub of water with a cup of apple cider vinegar added, to restore and strengthen the acid mantle of the skin. Afterward, the body should be dried and rubbed briskly with a towel until a warm glow is felt.

Epsom Salt baths may also be used to help draw toxins out of the skin. These baths are especially beneficial if one is going through a "healing crisis" and is especially toxic. Such baths work best after the skin brushing and use of a loofah sponge. A tub is filled with warm water and four or more cups of Epsom Salt. This bath is quite relaxing, good for tense, sore muscles, and may be taken as often as needed.

Once a week for the first six months on the metabolic program, the patient should be rubbed from head to toe with a mixture of olive oil and castor oil in equal parts; then have a hot bath for 15 minutes to allow the oil to penetrate. This is followed by going to bed under heavy covers for about one hour to sweat toxins out, then by a cleansing shower.

One of the most effective means of detoxifying the body of radiation present in the environment because of nuclear power plants, industrial processes and atmospheric nuclear tests, is the salt and soda bath. One cup of sea salt and one cup of baking soda should be placed in a warm tub of water. A person should soak in this for 15 to 20 minutes. The head and hair should be immersed completely from time to time, and when finished, one should rinse under a warm shower. Taking this bath daily when the flu is going around will often increase one's resistance to the disease.

It is good to take this bath daily, for several days, after x-rays or any therapeutic radiation.

CHAPTER FOURTEEN

Structural Therapy and Cancer

Dr. Tedd Koren poses this question in *The American Chiropractor:* "What can chiropractic do for cancer?" He provides the answer: "Absolutely nothing."[1]

Dr. Koren expounds upon his thoughts on the relationship between chiropractic and malignancy. "The answer to 'what can chiropractic do for any disease?' is 'nothing.' Because chiropractic doesn't address itself to diseases, but to dis-ease. The question must be interpreted and answered in the light of an understanding of chiropractic.

"The question is really: 'Can an organism that is physiologically sound, that is operating free from dis-ease, that has no nerve interference, do anything for cancer?' The answer is 'Yes.'

"Cancer is like any other disease, in that the individual's level of resistance plays a major role in the disease's etiology and prognosis. Nerve interference causes a body to function in a state less than its physiological optimum. . . . In order to have high resistance, you need a body free of nerve interference. . . . A body that is functioning normally will be in a better position to check any abnormal functions within it—cancer included."[2]

Structural therapies—chiropractic, osteopathy, cranial osteopathy, mandibular equilibration, spinal column stressology, reflexology and massage—are believed by many metabolic physicians to be the most underrated of the powerful weapons in the arsenal against cancer. Part of current medicine's dubious legacy to modern man, these physicians feel, is an overinfatuation with the biochemical aspects of health, at the expense of the structural, emotional and spiritual aspects. Even the mental aspects of healing are generally more accepted by the medical establishment than the structural aspects. Medical doctors have, it is felt, basically attempted to freeze structurally-oriented physicians out of the healing community, in apparent defiance of the axiom that "function follows form." Because of the general reluctance of most medical doctors to accept the value of chiropractors and other structural therapists, chiropractors have formed a healing community that is essentially their own, one characterized by an appreciation of natural healing modalities and immune function.

People with cancer who are on a metabolic program are advised by metabolic doctors to see one or more types of structural therapists on a regular basis. It is often advised that cancer patients, whose emotionally and biochemically stressed and imbalanced bodies are considered to be equally overburdened structurally, see a chiropractor almost every week during the first few months of their program. They may be advised by the chiropractor to come more or less often.

For a person whose physical existence is hanging in a fine balance between health and disintegration, this structural therapy is often considered to be enough to tip the balance toward health.

Chiropractic and Health Stimulation

Most people have only a limited appreciation of the possible benefits that can be derived from chiropractic; many consider it little more than an elevated form of massage for a sore back. Chiropractic, though, is a system of direct physical manipulation of nerves, muscles, tissues and bones, in an attempt, primarily, to achieve proper nerve function. Every biochemical action in the body is dependent upon nerve stimulation, and the degree of proper nerve function will, to a large extent, govern the degree of efficiency of the biochemical processes. "Chiropractic," writes Julius Dintenfass, D.C., "considers the implications of the neuro-muscular-skeletal mechanisms of the body as having a prime priority in the regulation and integration of the body changes to maintain homeostasis. The central control of these mechanisms is located within the cerebro-spinal-vertebral complex of the body."[3]

Implicit in the attempt to establish proper neurological function is a belief that if proper nerve function is achieved, the body will be able to defeat disease. Structural therapists believe that disease is a combination of health insults from outside the body, biochemical imbalances, and a lack of proper integration, or "teamwork," among organs and glands. Both of the two latter conditions can be caused by lack of proper nerve communication among organs and glands. "The concept of disease as resulting from integrative disorders," writes Dr. John Mason in *Perspectives in Biology and Medicine,* "rather than local or regional disorders, seems worthy of serious consideration on both theoretical and clinical grounds, particularly now that neuroendocrine systems provide new perspective, because of their linking of the brain and all somatic tissues."[4]

"Chiropractic," writes Dr. Dintenfass, "considers not only the local problem of the patient, but views the patient in a larger sense, because of the interaction of one part of the body with all other parts."[5]

This belief in the necessity of proper organ and glandular "teamwork" fits perfectly with the metabolic physicians' perspectives of health and disease. Just as a therapy program needs to address all of the body's organs and glands, so also, they feel, is structural therapy needed to help each organ and gland contribute its share, in a nerve-orchestrated, symbiotic symphony of health. "Chiropractic," says R. J. Quinlan, D.C., "is the clinical science of applying measured amounts of force, in specific vectors, to cause a beneficial alteration in the structure. The desire for alteration in a deranged structure, without interference, allowing normal conductivity, and thus providing the specific individual tissues it enervates with the proper amount of nervous energy is the force that sustains life."[6]

This stimulation of neurological function, then, is thought

to be helpful for healthy persons, people with cancer, and people with other pathologies. Professional chiropractic journals regularly report evidence of structural therapy benefitting patients with cancer, arthritis, Parkinson's disease, fatigue, backache, hypertension, allergies, facial nerve disorders, emotional instability, migraine headaches and numerous other ailments.

Chiropractic and Cancer

Chiropractic appears to help the cancer patient through two mechanisms: (1) improving neurological function of nerves traveling to organs and glands specifically associated with immunity to cancer, such as the thymus or liver, and (2) improving general energy levels and systemic recuperative potential.

Chiropractors, among their other functions, correct "subluxations," or misalignments of spinal-column vertebrae that create nerve blockage to specific glands and organs. Chiropractors are often able to pinpoint which nerves exit the spinal column at which vertebrae, and are thus able to know if a particular subluxation might be creating a problem in a distant part of the body. When they are able to correct the subluxation, they restore proper nerve stimulation to the impaired area. If the impaired area includes an organ or gland that is vital to the body's anti-cancer mechanisms, such as the pancreas, liver or thymus, resistance to cancer can increase dramatically following chiropractic adjustment. Metabolic doctors have observed this phenomenon many times.

Jerry Whigman, D.C., of Detroit, recently reported in the *Digest of Chiropractic Economics* that he believes chiropractic adjustment, when applied with a proper metabolic program, is the most important facet of helping patients overcome uterine cancer. Dr. Whigman says that, to fight cancer, the primary emphasis should be on stimulating proper nerve function of the organs of "digestion, absorption, assimilation and elimination."[7]

This stimulation of specific organs and glands to combat cancer is commonly done by a great many chiropractors. Because they are not licensed to "treat" cancer, however, they must be prudently circumspect about their public acknowledgement of the important role that chiropractic can play in resistance to cancer.

The other benefit of chiropractic to cancer patients—improving the entire system's recuperative potential—is no less important than chiropractic's more specific benefits. Most metabolic programs are, of course, based on the concept that the entire body, not just a few major organs and glands, is needed to fight malignancy.

Full Spinal Therapies

Structural therapies that are similar to conventional chiropractic are the "full-spinal" therapies. Full spinal therapies are approaches that treat the spinal column as a unit, rather than treating individual parts of it. One of the most advanced full-spinal therapies is "spinal column stressology," which was created by Lowell Ward, D.C., of Long Beach, California.

Dr. Ward originated the theory that a misaligned or displaced spinal column not only reflects stress put upon the body, but creates stress as well. He believes that heavy stress on the body, whether it's emotional, nutritional, traumatic or congenital, will cause the spinal column as a whole to leave its proper position. Once out of its proper center of gravity, he believes, the "misplaced" spinal column will cause not only localized problems but also will drain the entire body of energy and health.[8]

Dr. Ward is the originator of the perception of the spinal column as a "singular, synchronous, functional unit."[9] Most health practitioners, he says, view the spinal column in terms of localized, isolated problems, without taking into account the fact that all misalignments create reactions elsewhere in the spinal column, a process he calls "synchronicity."[10]

Dr. Ward combines the concept of synchronicity and the view of the spinal column as a single unit to arrive at the theory that health is utterly dependent upon the total, full-length spinal column being in exactly the proper position and proper state of synchronicity. Any variance from this, he says, is not only a reflection of problems but a creator of them as well. The severity of variance reflects the severity (and also affects the severity) of the body's problems.[11]

When this condition occurs, says Dr. Ward, much more energy is needed merely to hold the body erect. Dr. Ward likens the condition to holding a bucket of water at arm's length, rather than the easily-maintained, normal position of straight down from the shoulders. How far the body is out of balance correlates to a measure he calls the "energy loss factor."[12]

Cancer, he believes, is one of the problems that results from a spinal column that is out of position. He believes that if the "energy loss factor" is severe, dysfunction of a number of systems that normally help resist cancer, including the immune, digestive and eliminative systems, may allow a condition favorable to malignant growth to occur.

"Degenerative diseases, including cancer, are often brought to the crisis stage by a failure of the immune system, which needs a strong supply of energy," says Dr. Ward. "The longer the body has to operate on inadequate energy, which it does in cases of spinal column displacement, the more it will deplete immunity, disrupt biochemical balance and wear down vital organs. Energy is the key to health. If you don't have it, you're dead; if it's reduced, you're sick. If it's abundant, you're healthy."[13]

Spinal column stressology and other full-spinal treatments have been proven to be very helpful for cancer patients. Doctors treating cancer patients frequently report seeing a renewed burst of energy in patients who undergo this therapy, followed by improvement in their condition of malignancy.

Holism and Chiropractic

Of essential importance, it is felt, in applying structural therapies to diseases like cancer, is using the treatment as part of a holistic, multi-faceted healing regime. Chiropractors, osteopaths or spinal column stressologists who myopically apply only their treatment to a condition as complex as malignancy are believed by metabolic doctors to be as likely to fail as are single-approach chemotherapists or radiologists.

The improved neurological function created by structural therapies are considered to be of limited value if complementary biochemical and mental therapies are not simultaneously applied. These other therapies are thought to bolster structural therapy as powerfully as structural therapy boosts them.

"Chiropractic," writes Dr. Dintenfass in the *Journal of Energy Medicine,* "considers the total person in relation to many environmental factors."[14]

"Permanent improvement requires a holistic approach," says Edward Guenette, D.C., co-founder of the Whole Health Institute of Leominster, Mass. "What we're dealing with is a question of the individual's basic resistance to stress, whether it be overwork, worry, a virus, bacteria or whatever. We must deal with the body's ability to 'hold' our chiropractic adjustments. A patient who gets no love, no tenderness and has a great deal of emotional stress, for instance, can come into my office every day and get an atlas alignment and return home feeling fine. But if we're going to talk about lasting change, then we have to talk about an all-around program of holistic health."[15]

Nutritional therapy is one of the most closely allied therapies to structural treatment, and is recommended by a great many structural therapists. "We have discovered," says Jack O. Taylor, D.C., "that patients following a nutritional program respond more rapidly to our structural therapy. We have also noted that patients with sound structures respond much more favorably to the nutritional therapy. While either therapy can be applied independently, maximum benefits are achieved when they are applied together.

"Nutrition causes a change in the function of the nervous system by supporting the structure, chemically creating an environment conducive to normal neuro-function—or by actually altering the cellular structure, molecularly enabling it to function more efficiently. Chiropractic-structural therapy causes a change in the nervous system's gross and molecular structure, thereby altering its function for the better."[16]

Many of the younger chiropractors are vitally interested in applying nutritional therapy as part of their services. One believer in the benefits of nutritional therapy is Dr. Duane Smith, a 32-year-old, Logan, Utah, graduate of the Palmer College of Chiropractic.

"When I was at Palmer they fed us a pretty 'straight' structural manipulation approach," he says. "But I went to every seminar I could, regardless of how experimental or crazy it sounded. I wanted to learn everything I could about the body. The more I learned, the more respect I gained for the body's own ability to recuperate. When I started practice I soon found out that manipulation alone just wasn't making it, so I experimented with a number of nutritional programs and supplements."[17]

Dr. Smith found that when he combined chiropractic with other naturalistic therapies, including nutrition, his results were improved.

Chiropractic, as a healing art, certainly does not exist in a vacuum. Dr. Tedd Koren asks, "Should a person who believes he has cancer go to a chiropractor, or to a medical doctor? That's a bad question. I believe the best answer would be twofold: (1) Chiropractic care should be included if a person doesn't receive medical care, so that the body will have the highest possible chance of fighting cancer. (2) If a person does receive medical care, he should go to a chiropractor to improve his nerve supply. . . ."[18]

Other Structural Therapies

Other structural therapies which are thought to be of possible benefit to the health of the cancer patient include osteopathy, cranial osteopathy, mandibular equilibration, massage, the Alexander and Feldenkrais methods, reflexology and bioenergetics.

Of these, osteopathy is the practice that is closest to the medical mainstream. Osteopathy is similar to chiropractic in its emphasis on using manipulative techniques to reverse biomechanical and neurological abnormalities. Osteopaths, unlike chiropractors, though, are also trained and licensed to fulfill all the functions of M.D.s. Osteopathic therapy can be fully as beneficial for cancer patients as chiropractic.[19]

Considered to be of even more benefit to many cancer patients is cranial osteopathy, a sub-specialty concerned with the neurological function of the skull. A total of 31 pairs of nerves emanate from the spine, while 12 pairs of nerves exit from the cranium.[20] These 12 pairs of cranial nerves are benefitted by cranial osteopathy, as is the cranial structure, which is composed of a series of bones that cranial therapists believe are subtly mobile. If these bones do not join together in proper balance and equilibrium, they are believed to cause undue direct pressure upon the brain and cranial nerves.

Included in the 12 pairs of cranial nerves are nerves that go to organs in the thoracic cavity, including the pancreas and organs of digestion. Improper function of these nerves is believed by metabolic doctors to be especially devastating to a cancer patient. Mandibular equilibration, discussed later in this chapter, also corrects cranial problems.

Reflexology is another excellent method of neurological stimulation that any individual can perform on himself or herself or that another member of the family can perform. There are also qualified professional reflexologists available throughout the country.

There are, according to reflexologists, nerve endings and "acupressure points" in the hands and feet "reflexing" to all organs of the body. Crystal-like formations, caused from lack of proper circulation, are believed to collect around these nerve endings and points, irritating them. Irritated points and endings in the hands and feet can cause problems in any part of the body.

As appropriate areas in the hands and feet are massaged, irritated endings receive better blood circulation. The increased circulation clears away the crystal-like formations. When this is accomplished, the areas are no longer irritated. As nerve function is normalized, unimpeded impulses again travel to the brain and various tissues, glands and organs. With balanced nerve impulses going into the various parts of the body, normal, healthy activity can, it is believed, once again take place.

Reflexology is a theory of stimulating organs and glands that anyone can learn. If the cancer patient or a member of the family is administering the reflexology, metabolic doctors recommend use of this therapy at least three times a week, or daily if possible. If a professional reflexologist is consulted, fewer treatments will be needed.

It is considered important that a cancer patient concentrate on stimulating first the pancreas and liver "pressure points," then those for any organs in which malignancy is present, and, thirdly, those for all remaining organs of the body.

Two excellent books on reflexology are: *Stories the Feet Can Tell* and *Stories the Feet Have Told,* by Eunice D. Ingham, P.O. Box 12642, St. Petersburg, Florida 33733, (813) 343-4811. Reflexology charts may be obtained from the same address.

Various forms of massage can eliminate muscular tensions, which can be a result of skeletal or emotional stress. This muscular tightness can also, it is believed, "lock in" stress. Cancer patients, in particular, may have integrated emotional stresses into their muscular make-up, as a response to fear of their disease. Massage, which, according to Dr. Robert Frager, can range from "sensual stroking to moderately painful digging into sore or tense muscles," stimulates circulation, relieves muscular tension and improves joint flexion.[21]

One type of massage believed to be especially helpful is shiatsu massage, which puts pressure upon the "acupressure points" of the body. "From centuries of clinical practice," says Dr. Frager, "shiatsu treatments have been successfully devised to relieve a wide variety of physical illnesses."[22]

The Alexander technique is a postural therapy that improves the body's natural balance, relieves muscular tension, and provides conservation of energy.[23] The Feldenkrais method also establishes more efficient use of the body, creating a greater sense of relaxation.[24] Bioenergetics is a series of techniques devised by Alexander Lowen, M.D., which facilitates removal of physical tensions and promotes deeper breathing.[25] None of these techniques, quite obviously, were designed or promoted as cancer therapies. They are, though, considered by metabolic physicians to be helpful for cancer patients. It has always been the aim of those using the metabolic approach to treat the patient who has the disease, rather than to treat the disease that has the patient.

Mandibular Equilibration

A final form of structural therapy, one that seems to be of special benefit to cancer patients, is the balancing of the lower jaw mechanism—the therapy of "mandibular equilibration." This therapy appears to provide to cancer patients benefits similar to those derived from cranial osteopathy—stimulation of the cranial nerves, which stimulate important organs in the thoracic cavity.

The lower jaw, the mandible, is allowed to move by two joints that meet the bones that make up the sides of the skull. These two ball-and-socket type joints allow the lower jaw to move freely in three dimensions: up and down, across, and in a gliding motion. The joints are called the "temporomandibular joints," or T.M.J.s.

The bones on the sides of the skull, the temporal bones, are also connected to the sphenoid bone, which forms the front of the skull. These bones are connected by a "knitted," suture joint. In all, there are 26 cranial bones, all connected with suture joints.

The nerves that connect the brain to the body come out of the base of the skull and run down the spinal column, and also come out of holes and canals in the sphenoid and the two temporal bones. These holes are called "foramina." Twelve pairs of cranial nerves exit the cranium through these foramina.

Some cranial nerves perform neurological functions in the head—the optic nerve goes to the eyes, for example, and the auditory nerve goes to the ear. But others travel to the trunk of the body; the vagus nerve, for example, leaves the brain through one of the foramina and, descending vertically along the side of the pharynx, goes all the way to the transverse colon. The vagus nerve partially controls breathing and swallowing, and carries fibers to the heart, digestive tract, respiratory tract, kidneys, liver, spleen and pancreas.

In a perfect cranial structure, the mandible is the seat of an impeccably aligned, balanced, tension-free construction of bones, muscles, ligaments and nerves. To be in perfect working order, the bones must be undamaged by trauma or malnutrition, the muscles and ligaments must be the proper length in relation to the bones, and the teeth must be healthy and functionally sound, erupted to their proper height and in balance with other teeth. In this ideal situation, the bones and muscles allow perfect nerve transmission.

The ideal situation is rare.

Many factors disrupt cranial perfection, including birth injury, accident, ill-fitting dentures and poor nutrition.

The result of misalignment and stress in the cranial structure is pressure on the foramina—the small holes or canals in the temporal and sphenoid bones through which the 12 pairs of cranial nerves leave the cranium. "If the bone that the nerve goes through is distorted, the nerve impulse transmission is disturbed," says Harris Kimbrough, D.D.S. of Algonquin, Illinois, perhaps the nation's top mandibular equilibration therapist. "Nerve transmission, with distorted sphenoid or temporal bones, can be either partially disturbed or radically disturbed, depending upon the degree of stress placed upon the individual foramen," says Dr. Kimbrough. "The temporomandibular joint is involved in 35 to 40 per cent of all neurological activity. Consequently, disruption of the T.M.J. mechanism has considerable neurological effects. Pressure on the vagus nerve, as it travels on its way to the organs of digestion, respiration and circulation, can be particularly harmful." Dr. Kimbrough corrects T.M.J. imbalance with a small acrylic device, called the "mandibular equilibration appliance," or M.E.A., which looks and is worn like a common tooth-straightening retainer. Patients wear this device for 6 to 12 months to correct T.M.J. problems.[26]

Metabolic physicians have seen many dramatic responses in cancer patients after they have undergone M.E.A. therapy. Not the least dramatic response was that of Dr. Kimbrough himself. Dr. Kimbrough had a presumably "incurable" form of cancer, and was losing ground in his struggle against it, even though he was on a strict metabolic program. When he was fitted with his M.E.A., though, his improvement was sudden, and eventually total. He has since devoted his life to working with the M.E.A.

The Relative Importance of Various Structural Therapies

Because of the scarcity of some of the specialists who apply these techniques, most patients are not able to undergo all the structural therapies that might help.

In light of this, the therapies have been rated in order of what most metabolic doctors consider descending importance to the cancer patient. Because of their synergistic and interrelated qualities, certain of the therapies can most effectively be engaged in simultaneously. In order of benefit, the therapies are:

1. Cranial osteopathy and mandibular equilibration.
2. Full spinal chiropractic adjustments and mandibular equilibration.
3. Osteopathic manipulations and mandibular equilibration.
4. Cranial osteopathy.
5. Full spinal chiropractic adjustments.
6. Osteopathic manipulations.
7. Chiropractic adjustments (less than full spinal).
8. Reflexology treatments, various forms of massage, and various forms of postural integration.

People who are ill should keep "shopping" for structural therapists until they find one they feel they receive substantial benefit from. Not all practitioners are equally beneficial to all patients.

Structural therapies, like many of the detoxification techniques, can provide real pleasure and almost immediate improvement in comfort and well-being. These therapies should not be neglected. Indeed, metabolic doctors tell patients that these therapies should be used, enjoyed and learned from.

CHAPTER FIFTEEN

The Emotional and Spiritual Aspects of Cancer

Cancer can be a blessing. Many cancer patients have said that to their metabolic physicians. Cancer can compel one to forge one's physical habits into a lifestyle more in accord with nature, and thus cause one to eventually glean more energy from life than had been possible before the "rude awakening" of cancer. More important than this physical reawakening, though, is the emotional and spiritual rebirth that is often a part of recovery from cancer. This renaissance of peace and hope is so closely tied to regaining health that many metabolic doctors have come to believe that recovery might not be possible without it.

For many years, holistic health practitioners who included a mental/spiritual component in their therapies were sneered at by many members of the mechanistic medical community as being unscientific faith-healers, charlatans who merely played upon the placebo effect. Almost no differentiation was made between the most scientific mind/body practitioners and the most cynical tent-meeting fakers who made bogus "cripples" toss down their crutches and walk. In the late 1960s and 1970s, though, perhaps because of a general rekindling of interest in spiritualism, and because of the unprecedented popularity of various forms of psychological therapy, the stigma attached to mind/body healing receded.

Currently, even the most technologically-infatuated practitioners are having to admit that the mind, embodying one's psychological and spiritual beliefs, is of paramount importance in one's physical health. Doctors who stubbornly deny that the mind plays a vital role in health are now becoming as isolated from the mainstream as were mind/body healers in earlier decades.

All good metabolic programs contain a psychological/ spiritual component. Indeed, for many patients, metabolic doctors say, the program would be an unmitigated failure if this element were not addressed.

For some people, the psychological aspect is believed to be of more importance than the spiritual aspect. For others, the inverse is true. A complete metabolic patient evaluation procedure can ascertain a person's degree of spiritual peace and psychological strength by asking many questions about these areas. If there seem to be problems in either area, as there often are, particularly in people who may have been told they are terminally ill, metabolic doctors generally advise the patient to seek the help of their choice and to put their own energy into excising psychological and spiritual uneasiness. The methods that patients use to try to solve their problems are, of course, numerous. Their successes are varied. Those who do succeed, though, often eventually consider their disease to have been a blessing. Sometimes they feel blessed by having cancer even when they do not recover, as remarkable as that may seem.

The Psychology of Cancer

What comprises the connection between mind and body is not obvious. It is a connection that has one end in the physical realm, the body, and one in the non-physical realm, the world of abstract thought. Writers, theologians, philosophers and scientists have grappled with the nature of the mind/body relationship for ages.

In a purely physical sense, we know that the brain is connected to the nervous system through the spinal cord and cranial nerves, that the nervous system is connected to the endocrine and limbic and the immune systems, that those systems are connected to the internal organs, that the organs, through blood and lymphatic fluid, are connected to all bodily tissues, that the tissues are formed of cells, and that cells are formed of molecules. But this doesn't tell us very much about the paths of communication and control. There is no single "highway" in the body, no single "telephone line" or "airwave" which could be considered the definitive connection between body and mind. Consequently, almost all forms of medicine that have tried to bridge the physical and non-physical realms, be they Oriental medicines or Western explorations of psychosomatics, have often been regarded with skepticism by mechanistic, physical-based physicians.

Nonetheless, the mind-body connection, however mysterious, is currently being utilized for the treatment of, among other ailments, cancer. Cancer therapist O. Carl Simonton, M.D. is currently the leading pioneer in this endeavor. He is using psychological techniques to influence regression of cancer. He has been doing this for about ten years and his results have been outstanding. A large number of therapists around the country are now using Dr. Simonton's methods, which they generally combine with physical cancer therapies.

Laboratory Experiments

It has long been thought that mental/emotional states play a part in whether or not a person contracts cancer, and in how well he or she responds to treatment.

The Greek physician Galen said almost two thousand years ago that cancer was due in part to "a melancholy disposition."[1] The English physician Sir James Paget wrote a century ago that "The cases are so frequent in which deep anxiety, deferred hope and disappointment are quickly followed by the growth and increase of cancer that we can hardly doubt mental depression is a weighty additive to the cancer condition."[2]

In 1846, Englishman W. A. Walshe observed that "mental disquietude" played a part in cancer development; he advised people with cancer in their family history to avoid stressful occupations.[3] Between 1885 and 1900 Parker, Watson and Snow published papers that showed a connection between marital and emotional stress, depression and cancer.[4] At this time, though, there was no science of psychology, so little was done with these studies.

In the mid-1950s, a rebirth of interest occurred in the

theory that cancer is partially caused by the emotions. Since then, about 200 articles about it have been written, many of which are reports of original research. Of the 200 articles, not one concludes that there is no relationship between cancer and the emotions.[5]

Much of the research has tried to prove the premise that stress decreases a person's ability to resist cancer. Other research has dealt with predicting onset of cancer by studying an individual's personality traits.

Stress and Resistance to Cancer

It is believed by most doctors that a strong immune system can fight off malignant cell growth, usually before any visible symptoms appear. It is further believed that stress weakens the immune system.

Researcher Vernon Riley reported in 1975 that he was able to alter the incidence of breast cancer in mice from 92 percent in stressful conditions to 7 percent in a protected, non-stressful environment. He said that over-activation of the adrenal glands from stress resulted in impairment of the thymus in mice, and led to an impairment of the immune mechanisms.[6]

G. F. Soloman and A. A. Amkraut reported, in 1972, that in an experiment on rabbits, induced lesions in specific portions of the hypothalamus, the part of the brain most closely associated with emotions, impaired the rabbits' production of antibodies and made them less able to dispel malignant tissue grafted onto them. Stimulation of the same area had the opposite effect.[7]

R. C. LaBarba reported in 1970 that stress in the form of electric shock invariably led to the early appearance of mammary tumors in cancer-prone mice. He also noted that overcrowding of mice led to early cancers. LaBarba reviewed all the existing literature, both American and foreign, about stress/malignancy animal experiments, and found that all of it agreed that stress facilitated the onset and growth of cancer. The theory most often cited as explanation for this was that stress inhibited growth of antibodies, disturbed the hormonal balance and cellular metabolism, and upset the endocrine system.[8] All of these physical disturbances have been linked to cancer in numerous other experiments.

No researcher was able to prove which physical factors that are affected by the nervous system are the most important in immunity to malignancy; probably a delicate, vast and complicated interrelationship is the key to resistance.

What is more apparent is that, no matter how difficult it is to define the nature of the stress-disease link, such a link does exist.

Personality Traits as Cancer Predictors

T. H. Holmes developed in 1970 a scale for humans that associates stressful events with illness. Holmes identified 43 "life change events," and, by interviewing, was able to rate them in importance. The event regarded as most serious was death of a spouse; the least serious "life change event" was arrest for a minor violation. Holmes compared these events to onset of disease in individuals. It was shown that the degree of importance and accumulation of life-changes was accompanied by a corresponding vulnerability to illness, including cancer.

A 1977 study at Texas A&M University by Drs. W. R. Smith and Henry Sebastian showed that cancer patients tested had had almost twice the number of emotionally upsetting experiences in their lives as a control group. The researchers said the experiment was "powerfully supportive of the theory that emotions and cancer are linked."[10]

If one accepts that stress is a precursor to disease, including cancer, then it stands to reason that certain stressful experiences and stress-burdened personalities should be predictive of cancer. Many studies support this idea.

Dr. Lawrence LeShan presented in 1966 results of a 12-year study of 450 cancer patients who were given extensive psychological testing. The following pattern of life history emerged in 72 percent of the cancer patients, compared to 10 percent of a control group: During the first seven years, the child had difficulty relating to others, often because of loss of a parent or sibling, and usually blamed himself or herself for the problems. In adulthood, problems with relationships took the form of a strong attachment to one person, with all the tensions inherent in such a strong, single relationship emerging. LeShan found four characteristics common to cancer patients: (1) loss of an important relationship prior to diagnosis of cancer, (2) inability to express hostility, (3) tension over the death of a parent, often in the distant past, and (4) a basic attitude of helplessness and hopelessness.[11]

C. B. Thomas and K. R. Duszynski reported in 1974 that a lack of closeness to parental figures was higher in cancer patients than in mentally ill patients or eventual suicides.[12]

A. H. Schmale and H. K. Iker reported in 1971 that they thought women with a "helpless prone personality" would be likely to develop cancer. They psychologically tested a group of healthy women who had suspicious PAP smears, and were able to predict eventual malignancy with a degree of accuracy of 73.6 percent. E. M. Blumberg did extensive psychological testing of cancer patients in 1954 and found that patients with fast growing tumors were characteristically more defensive, had a stronger desire to appear good, had more tension from emotional conflicts, and were less able to defend against anxiety than a group with slow-growing tumors. During a second phase of the study, these criteria were used as predictors of cancer and were proven correct in 78 percent of subjects tested.[13]

Researcher B. Klopfer also contrasted people with fast and slow growing tumors and found that those whose tumors grew fastest were most likely to try hard to be good and loyal, to defend their egos, and to be tightly bound to a concrete, inflexible approach to reality. Klopfer used these criteria as predictors of cancer and achieved 80 percent accuracy.[14]

W. A. Greene reported in 1966 results of a 15-year study of the psychological and social experiences of patients developing leukemia and lymphoma. Of 16 male patients studied, all were experiencing loss or separation from a mother or mother-figure during initial onset of the disease. Of 32 female patients, 30 developed symptoms in the wake of separation from an important love object. In another study of 61 male patients, 57 were adjusting to separation losses, most often separation from a job.[15]

J. I. Wheeler and B. M. Caldwell reported in 1955 that women they psychologically tested, who had breast cancer or cervical cancer, had been less responsive than average in their sexual relations. A 1952 survey by C. L. Bacon and others showed that women with breast cancer showed a higher tendency toward sexual inhibition and frustration than even women with diagnosed neuroses. These women were characteristically excessively pleasant and could not deal with anger.[16]

Dr. Lawrence LeShan has probably looked harder and longer into the emotional causation of cancer than any other researcher. He states, in *You Can Fight for Your Life,* "There is a general type of personality configuration among the majority of cancer patients."[17] That configuration, generally speaking, is of a person who has had an emotionally difficult life, who has responded by withdrawing from negative emotions, and who, generally, even if it isn't always obvious, views life from a perspective of "helplessness and hopelessness."

Which leads to a larger question.

What can be done about it?

Emotional Therapy for Cancer Patients

Intervention is the next step.

The immune response, it would appear, can be stimulated by psychological therapy, which practitioners say can be not only cancer-preventive but also therapeutic. This therapy involves freeing the mind of stress, and channeling energy into positive thoughts.

Dr. O. Carl Simonton, radiologist, major in the U.S. Army and University of Oregon Medical School graduate, is the leader in this endeavor.

"My training and thinking about cancer were standard through the first half of my training," writes Dr. Simonton, now director of the Cancer Counseling and Research Center in Fort Worth, Texas, in *Getting Well Again.* "I didn't think a particular attitude mattered. Sometimes patients would say, 'Oh doctor, I've got so much faith in you and the machines you're using! I really believe in them!' And I'd think, 'I don't give a damn if you believe or don't believe.'

"I first came to change when I was introduced to the surveillance theory, which became widely accepted in the 1960s. Assuming that theory, which says you periodically have malignant cells but destroy them naturally through your immune system, I no longer was burdened with destroying every single cancer cell through radiation. Before I accepted that, I didn't appreciate that cancer waxes and wanes, like diabetes or arthritis. I'd thought cancer had, without outside interference, a completely downhill pattern.

"I was also influenced by the advent of biofeedback. The concept that we can influence our blood pressure, blood flow, heart rate, skin temperature, etc., just by thinking about them while watching a monitoring device, was intriguing. It didn't seem like too big a step to begin influencing the basic defense system.[18]

"Freud addressed this. He said that if we were to really address ourselves to the emotional needs of the masses, it would have to be through some form of hypnosis or self-hypnosis. The methods we now use—guided imagery, autogenic training, active imagination, mediation, Jacobson's progressive relaxation techniques—are all closely allied with self-hypnosis.

"In Portland, Oregon, the day came when I had to do something with all these thoughts. I sat down with one of my radiology patients and explained to him about progressive relaxation and guided imagery. He was a 61-year-old man with advanced throat cancer, down to 91 pounds—he couldn't swallow and was going downhill fast. I thought it might help and hoped it wouldn't hurt.

"I had him image his white cells attacking cancer cells. He had a dramatic response. The cancer disappeared. My associate said it was the first time he'd ever seen this type and stage of cancer respond. He sailed through therapy. That was over six years ago and he still has no sign of cancer. He used the same technique on his arthritis and it stopped; he used it on sexual impotence that he'd had for 20 years and began having normal relations.

"This kind of blew the back of my head off.

"It was very difficult for me to understand. What was even more difficult was to see how many other patients refused to do it. Hell, I'm the big cancer specialist—they're supposed to do just what I tell them, aren't they? But many refused.

"As I began to tàlk to them I began to appreciate that in all of us is a will to live and a will to die. In the imaging process one comes to terms with the will to live and die. Out of all this developed the psychotherapeutic approach—it grew from trying to understand why a gravely ill person would not take 15 minutes to try to get well.''[19]

Fifteen minutes of imaging, three times a day, is the core of the Simonton therapy. During that time the patient, who is probably undergoing simultaneous physical treatment, relaxes his or her body as much as possible, then tries to picture the white blood cells of the immune system fighting the cancer cells. The imaging should be as vivid and active as the patient can make it. Patients frequently imagine their white blood cells are sharks and their cancer cells are helpless victims.

Many patients have difficulty imagining their white blood cells defeating their cancer cells. Sometimes this is because they don't think they will be able to overcome cancer. This is a manifestation of the ''helpless and hopeless'' personality. Often the patient who is experiencing difficulty imaging discovers for the first time that he or she has mixed feelings about the disease —in some ways, he or she wants to be sick. At this point enters the other part of the Simonton therapy—emotional counseling.

Dr. Simonton believes most cancer patients have unconsciously—ocassionally consciously—allowed themselves to get cancer when they could have stopped it. For many people, cancer has good side-effects: a neglected wife is no longer neglected, an overworked man can relax, a person with repressed anger can have something to be angry about. There are as many reasons for wanting to be sick as there are unmet needs. Dr. Simonton calls these the ''secondary gains'' of the disease.[20]

Also, there are many people who don't necessarily want to be sick, but because of emotional problems, inadvertently block the health-maintaining flow of energy and physical exchange from system to system.

Dr. Simonton believes that the same mechanisms that seem to induce cancer—mind to nervous system, to limbic system, to endocrine system, to immune system, etc.—can also be used to reverse cancer.[21]

Consequently, Dr. Simonton believes that a person must accept personal responsibility for the disease in order to begin reversing it. This does not necessarily mean ''blame'' in the negative sense—a person who is taught to repress anger and is rewarded for being cheerful throughout life, at the expense, perhaps, of developing an ulcer or malignancy, is not blameworthy, only misdirected.

Taking responsibility for one's own direction does, however, necessarily imply having the power to change it. Hence, responsibility takes on a meaning of freedom. Having no responsibility means one is a victim, without power or influence.

Often the medical profession, family and peers reinforce the feeling that the cancer patient is a helpless victim.[22] Teeth-gritting passivity and cooperation with "authorities" is generally considered laudable behavior from a cancer patient.

Stephanie Matthews Simonton, Dr. Simonton's wife and colleague, is in charge of the emotional counseling at the center. "The work we do," she says, "is only with people who believe they emotionally participated in their disease and want to explore it. We try to help them discover a meaning for their disease. We have them look at the events and lifestyles six to 18 months to two years before onset of symptoms, to see what they can learn about why their defenses broke down. This is the hardest stage for a patient. They have to get a feeling for what they were doing, so they don't feel like a helpless victim.

"The second stage," says Stephanie Simonton, "is to look at the present life of a patient. What is the message of the disease to their current life? The disease can have a purposeful meaning. One man who spent his life taking care of others said the message of his disease was for him to learn to take care of himself.

"The hardest part is for the patient not to feel blame and guilt when they see how they participated. Our society is in many ways geared toward making us participate in the causing of the disease—we're so often rewarded for putting our own emotional needs last. We're taught that we needn't feel guilty about filling our stomachs when we're hungry, but we do feel guilty about filling our emotional needs.

"A regression in the illness can be a good learning experience. We teach patients to remember their activities on the day they needed more painkillers—who they talked to, what they did.

"You can't generalize about what a person needs—only he or she knows."[24]

Patients often find that they respond well to the imaging techniques when they have good reasons to live and respond poorly when they don't. Dr. Simonton has patients make lists of what they want from life—pleasure goals, work goals, relationship goals, both short-term and long-term. They are encouraged to fulfill these goals and are helped to overcome obstacles preventing fulfillment. The counselors help patients deal with family members, peers and employers who stand in the way of the patient's having a meaningful life.

The crux of the counseling is helping the patient dispel feelings of helplessness and hopelessness, teaching him or her to discharge negative emotions, and helping the patient learn to live the particular life he or she really wants to live.

With this groundwork laid, patients try to rally their immune defenses with the relatively simple imaging techniques.

Most cancer patients, Dr. Simonton has found, cannot accept these ideas, nor are they able to do the imaging. Accepting the responsibility for the disease and actively taking part in treatment does not appeal to most cancer patients. "People will go to any length to have someone else heal them," says Stephanie Simonton. "Our patients are the ones who are in control. We aren't the healers."[25] The center gets several hundred calls per month from cancer patients, but only about 150 per year go through the therapy.

Of those who undergo the therapy, the success rate is very encouraging. Dr. Simonton, in *Getting Well Again,* details the results of the 159 stage-four, or terminal, patients he treated over a seven-year period. Of those 159, none of whom were expected to live longer than a year, 63 are still alive, 76 are dead, and 20 were unavailable for follow-up. Of the living patients, 22 percent had no evidence of disease, 19 percent had regressing tumors, 27 percent had a stabilized disease, and 32 percent had some new tumor growth. Of the living patients, 51 percent were working full-time, 25 percent were working half-time, and only 3 percent were hospitalized.[26]

The recovery statistics for patients in earlier stages of cancer are higher, but most patients so far have used the Simonton method only as a last resort. Attitude, however, is considered more important than stage of disease.[27]

Patients can learn the therapy at the center. They can also learn it on their own, by listening to tapes available from the center. More buy tapes than attend the center's program. Other physicians, such as Emmett Miller, M.D., of Palo Alto, California, (415) 328-7171, provide excellent healing-oriented tapes.

Non-cancer patients can also benefit from the techniques as a cancer prevention measure, according to the executive director of the center, Bill Morton. One of the tapes deals with health in general.

"It takes a special type of person to make this therapy work," says Morton. "The patients must be highly motivated, intelligent and flexible. The patients must be responsible for themselves.

"What we don't want," he says, "is for someone to waltz in and expect Dr. Simonton to lay hands on them."[28]

Although Dr. Simonton is the acknowledged leader in the field, he is by no means the country's only mind/body cancer therapist. He and his associates have personally trained a large number of physicians and psychologists, who practice throughout the nation, and other doctors have read his work and employ his methods. Psychological therapists other than those associated with Dr. Simonton are also working with cancer patients. These therapists employ a wide variety of techniques, including talk counseling, bodywork, primal-based therapies, and psychoanalysis.

Whomever the patient feels most comfortable with is the correct therapist for that patient.

Spiritualism and Cancer

Many metabolic doctors feel that spiritual attitudes are no less important than the emotions in relation to cancer. It is even more difficult to quantify the effects of spiritual attitudes, however, than it is to quantify the effects of emotional attitudes. Clearly, nothing is more ethereal, and therefore more difficult to integrate with our current mechanistic concepts of science, than religion and spiritualism. Also, no subject is more likely to arouse contentiousness than is religion.

Nonetheless, the personal experiences of many metabolic doctors with many patients have led the doctors to believe that patients who are most at peace with the universe and their role in it are most likely to recover from cancer. And for patients who are not able to recover, a secure sense of spiritual linkage to existence appears to provide immense comfort.

The difference between spiritual peacefulness and emotional peacefulness depends mostly upon where the patient feels the peace has come from. "The basic difference between religious healing and (emotional healing) is the insistence on the part of those who do the healing, and usually on the part of those who are healed, that the power comes directly from God or from divine sources, and that both healer and recipient of the healing are merely instruments of that divine will," writes Professor Hans Holzer, in *Beyond Medicine.*[29] Holzer also points out that "true religious healing requires no intermediary gifted with extraordinary powers."[30]

The histories of virtually all religions include innumerable accounts of miraculous healings, which appear in many cases to be not only verifiable, but also inexplicable as either a physical or even a psychological reaction. The history of Christianity includes accounts of miraculous healings before, during and after the time of Christ, including literally hundreds which have appeared to have occurred at the French grotto of Lourdes. Among these was one directly witnessed by Dr. Alexis Carrell, the man who created the "artificial heart." A malignant lesion dried up before the doctor's eyes and fell off the patient's hand in a matter of moments.[31] One can, of course, choose to debunk this incident as a form of trickery, as well as that of every other example of faith healing that has occurred over the millenia.

Whether the admittedly amazing results gained by faith healing are, as Hans Holzer writes, "achieved by intellectual means, by experimental means, or by the invocation of divine powers, is really beside the point. The fact remains that religious healing works often enough to make it a responsible form of unorthodox healing."[32]

Spirit as Life

"When a man dies," philosopher Charles Peguyh wrote,

"he does not die of the disease he has, he dies of his whole life."[33] It seems absurd to many metabolic doctors to try to disconnect from a person's "whole life" his or her spiritual life. This artificial dissection, convenient though it may be for certain physicians, psychologists or spiritualists, flies in the face of common sense.

The best approaches from the history of the healing tradition, many metabolic doctors feel, were those that treated the patient as a triumvirate of mind, body and spirit. In fact, prior to the rise of the Industrial Revolution and the phase of technological medicine that this Revolution ushered in, these approaches were more the rule than the exception. In the early days of most cultures' medicines, writes historian Robert McKechnie, M.D., "medicine and religion were one."[34]

Dr. McKechnie states that "psychosomatic medicine became the first established branch of medicine. . . . Only in the last 200 years or so did the physician begin to turn away from the semi-mystic thinking that governed his profession for so many years."[35]

This abandonment of spiritualism may have installed the doctor as the high priest of technological medicine, but it does not, in many cases, appear to serve the best interests of the patient. It often seems to work against patients for a simple reason: patients who address their spiritual malaise generally appear to, in the opinions of metabolic doctors, feel better, and be more prone to recover from their diseases.

Patients' Responses to Spiritualism

Many patients reportedly resist admitting that they feel spiritual unrest, just as they often resist changing emotionally. Eydie Mae, who recovered from cancer with the metabolic Gerson therapy, writes of her unwillingness to change her spiritual belief system during the course of her illnes: "In the past we had placed the hard core Bible believers in the realm of dreamers, or fairy tale believers, or deluded extremists. . . ."[36]

Forced by her disease to examine with profound seriousness her entire set of religious beliefs, she found her own doubts to be ultimately, for her, untenable. "After wrestling with our studies, our minds, and our prejudices, many of our former doubts and delusions have been cleared up. . . ." She finally decided that she did believe in a divine entity, and said,

"I am no longer afraid to die. My questions about the future have been answered. . . ."[36]

She found that accepting death released her from many fears and replenished her appreciation of life. This, in turn, she felt, significantly expedited her healing.

Supposedly terminal cancer patient Dore Deverell lived to write about a similar experience. "If you don't like the idea of God," she advises cancer patients," and could care less about asking Him for anything, just keep realizing that deep within you is all knowledge." She reports feeling "freedom and joy" when she began to believe in the concept that she was inextricably tied to the universe, and that her physical mortality did not necessarily limit her role in a greater existence.

Dr. W. D. Kelley, in seminars with doctors, often describes his own spiritual change. At one seminar he said: "In my own experience with cancer, I found that accepting death as an integral part of life, and not as a definition of existence's finiteness, was of the utmost importance. As long as I resisted the idea of death, as long as I asked God, 'Why me?' I was burdened with a feeling of life's shortness and was shackled by fear. But when I let go of my desperate attachment to life, I found that there was still life in me, and that there would continue to be up until the moment of my passage, and that I had no good reason not to draw as much from this life as possible. When I began acting upon this revelation, the outward flow of energy from my being began to reverse itself. I began taking in energy that was greater than the energy that left my body, and I began to heal.

Spiritual Guidelines

Many metabolic doctors recommend to patients variations of the following general guidelines. Having made these recommendations, they invariably then leave to the patient the choice of which spiritual path to take.

These general guidelines often include the following:

1. One should accept the fact that he or she is afflicted with only a symptom of ill health, a malignant tumor, and that recovery is possible.

2. One should establish a faith in a power greater than

oneself, and know that with the help of one's God, one can regain health and harmony.

3. One should make the decision to turn his or her will and his or her life over to the care of one's God.

4. One should conduct a complete self-analysis to better understand one's spiritual beliefs.

5. One should admit to one's God and to himself or herself the exact nature of what one finds to be one's shortcomings.

6. One should be willing to give up what he or she is doing wrong.

7. One should seek through prayer or meditation to improve conscious contact with one's God. One should pray for knowledge about divine will, and for the strength to carry out this will.

8. Having had a spiritual awakening as a result of these principles, one should practice these principles in daily thoughts and actions.

Several other guidelines for people who are critically ill are offered by Harold Bloomfield, M.D., in *Health and Happiness.* These include:

1. Face and accept the reality of your own death.
2. Accept the responsibility for your own happiness.
3. Develop balance and harmony.
4. Face your weaknesses and grow.
5. Spend time alone.
6. Read about spiritual growth.
7. Strengthen your religious ties.
8. Don't be hesitant to ponder the big unanswered questions of life.
9. Beware of the belief that you can ever stop growing.[39]

Patients are advised by most metabolic physicians simply to examine what is in their heads and hearts and souls, and to make peace with what is there.

Many people, especially those who develop cancer, feel that they are unworthy human beings, and that they have failed their families.

This is simply not true. It is a tragically misguided notion, and one that many metabolic physicians feel can be fatal for a cancer patient. Unlearning this fallacy can be, these physicians believe, a cancer patient's first giant step back towards life.

CHAPTER SIXTEEN

The Anti-Cancer Lifestyle

One of the most challenging tasks for the person who has cancer, and one most rich in rewards, is breaking up the harmful patterned habits that preceded the disease. Unless one's philosophy of life is bedrocked in a firm belief in the Fickle Finger of Fate, common sense compels one to realize that the lifestyle patterns that pre-dated the cancer probably played an integral role in its formation. Even the highest authorities at the National Cancer Institute now acknowledge that lifestyle errors account for up to 90 percent of all cancers.[1]

Paolo Mantegazza expresses the concept rather poetically: "Out of a hundred diseases, fifty are caused by our own faults, forty by our carelessness."[2]

"Lifestyle" commonly refers to one's diet, hygenic habits, physical activities, work habits, manner of dress, recreation, etc. In a broad sense, "lifestyle" encompasses a person's every frequently repeated action. But cancer patients, say metabolic doctors, need only be directly concerned with lifestyle factors that relate to disease causation. This chapter will discuss disease-related lifestyle factors which have not been previously examined in this book. This chapter will discuss the lifestyle factors of rest and relaxation, work, exercise, and smoking. These are the lifestyle factors, other than those mentioned elsewhere (such as diet or habitual exposure to chemicals) that a person with cancer are advised to be most concerned with. In most people with cancer, changes are recommended in these areas in order to guarantee recovery. Metabolic physicians report that patients who are unwilling to alter the living patterns that preceded their disease, which may also be keeping them from overcoming the disease, are patients who are quite literally threatening their own lives.

Changing Your Life

Most people who have cancer, say metabolic doctors, are people who have been, in a general sense, putting out more than they have been taking in. They are said to manifest this pattern in their relations with other people, in their work habits, in their nutritional habits, and even in their recreation. Through metabolic physicians' communications with thousands of people who have had cancer, it has been found that most people who contract cancer simply do not replenish their energy as quickly as they expend it. An extremely common occurrence is for a person with cancer to feel run-down and fatigued—mentally, emotionally and physically—for more than a year prior to onset of clinical symptoms of malignancy. In fact, metabolic physicians say that it is quite probable that severe, inexplicable fatigue is not only an early warning sign of cancer, but also a contributor to it.

Unfortunately, our society rewards people who indulge in over-stress and over-work, even though it scorns other forms of compulsive behavior, such as over-drinking or over-eating. The concept that one could overindulge in work is quite foreign to many of us. Our culture has decided that denial of one's basic need for rest and relaxation is somehow a virtue. We give each other "brownie points" for giving out more than we take in.

This self-denial of the need to rest and relax runs contrary to the laws of nature, and its reward is disease. We busy people can postpone systemic breakdown temporarily with symptom-suppressing drugs, surgical procedures, and stimulants, but as long as we "burn the candle at both ends," we are betting against the existence of a natural law of supply and demand—a bet which is, unfortunately, a "sucker's bet." Until America's population learns to follow the dictates of nature, say metabolic physicians, we will continue to be plagued with epidemics of degenerative diseases, including cancer. Joseph Pearce, in *Exploring The Crack in the Cosmic Egg,* says, "Consider one of the assumptions of Western rational scientism: the life force on our planet has evolved one of its most magnificent expressions, the human mind, the function of which is supposedly to outwit and dominate the life force from which it evolved."

Dr. Stanley Keleman writes that, "Man has gone through the stages of being a victim to nature, then dominating nature, and now trying to cooperate with nature."[4] Perhaps Dr. Keleman is a bit optimistic in his assumption that most people are now trying to cooperate with nature. Those who smoke cigarettes, overindulge in work, and fail to exercise, are swimming against the tide of nature, and will, in all likelihood, be dragged down by the undertow.

If cancer patients would just follow one rule, say many metabolic doctors, they would make the first movement towards recovery. The rule: "Be good to yourself."

Exercise

Exercise is an integral facet of the metabolic approach to cancer. Metabolic doctors recommend that exercise be pleasant and enjoyable. All lifestyle changes, they say, must afford more pleasure than pain, or they will not be continued. Pleasure may not come immediately from a lifestyle change, but if it does not come at all, the patient will revert to his or her old habits.

As long ago as 1911, according to O. Carl Simonton, M.D., prominent cancer researcher James Ewing observed that there was greater cancer incidence in the "indolent"[5] In 1921 Silvertsen and Dahlstrom studied the deaths of 86,000 cancer patients, and found that the death rate was highest among those whose work required the least muscular exertion.[6]

Dr. Simonton, whose anti-cancer program contains an exercise component, says in *Getting Well Again* that several animal experiments have shown that increased exercise causes enhanced resistance to cancer. He cites a 1938 experiment in which cancer-prone mice showed a decline of cancer incidence from 88 percent to 16 percent when they were exercised every day and their caloric intake was restricted.[7] H. P. Rusch and B. K. Kline observed similar reduction of tumor incidence when animals were exercised. Hoffman and Paschkis reported decreased tumor prowth, and sometimes disappearance of malignancy, in mice injected with an extract from mice who had been recently exercised and were fatigued.[8]

Exercise apparently has psychological as well as physical benefits. Dr. Simonton writes that "Exercise . . . produces significant psychological changes. . . . People on a regular exercise program . . . tend to be more flexible in their thinking and beliefs, they tend to have an increased sense of self-sufficiency, a strengthened self-concept, improved self-acceptance, less tendency to blame others, and less depression. The overall picture is that people engaged in regular exercise programs tend to develop a healthier psychological profile in general—one often identified with a favorable prognosis for the course of the malignancy."[9]

Aerobic exercise expert Dr. Kenneth Cooper believes that increased oxygen flow to the brain creates increased mental well-being.[10] Dr. Robert Brown of the University of Virginia believes that exercise is directly beneficial for depression.[11] Thaddeus Kostrubala, M.D., believes that running can sometimes cure some forms of mental illness.[12]

The physical benefits of exercise are many and varied, and can reportedly strengthen the other aspects of a metabolic program. Because the body's primary immune factors travel in the blood, the increased blood flow created by exercise is thought to be desirable for the cancer patient. Exercise also speeds the effects of a metabolic cancer program by accelerating all of the metabolic processes, including digestion, elimination and absorption of nutrients. The perspiration caused by many forms of exercise is considered a valuable addition to a cancer patient's detoxification program. Increased cellular oxygenation through added lung use is believed by metabolic doctors to directly influence reduction of tumor masses.

Exercise helps the entire system. Donald Ardell, Ph.D., writes that "exercise strengthens and improves the efficiency of the heart, blood vessels, and lungs; produces healthier body tissues, a better appestat mechanism, and a lower resting heart rate; facilitates increased lung capacity; reduces stored fat; and enables better digestion of food and more efficient elimination of waste."[13] Dr. Ancel Keyes reported that in a study of healthy young men required to stay in bed, there was general development of muscle atrophy, lost blood volume, loss of calcium, and a depletion in the muscle protein of potassium, several vitamins, phosphorus, sulphur, nitrogen and sodium.[14]

Arthur Kaslow, M.D., who has a self-care program for degenerative diseases, believes that the increased oxygenation caused by exercise is of vital importance in overcoming serious disease. He writes, "Oxygen is essential to all vital processes and is used by the body as it converts food into energy, builds and regenerates cells and tissue, and maintains homeostasis and balance."[15] The "revitalization" created by exercise, Dr. Kaslow says, "turns on the whole system and improves all body functions, changes attitudes, and stimulates new activities."[16]

Exercise is associated with virtually all societal longevity, including that of Russia's Hunzas and Ecuador's Vilcabamba Indians, who are believed to live to be 110 to 120 years of age. Britain's Thomas Paar, the man with the world's longest proven lifespan, did physical farm labor almost until the day of his death at age 152.[17]

Cancer patients are generally more able to exercise than is commonly believed. Dr. Simonton reports that over half of his patients who have been declared terminal are capable of the same amount of physical activity that they were before their disease. One patient with metastasized lung-kidney cancer, he reports, was able to complete a 26-mile marathon with no breathing problems.[18]

The only time exercise may be harmful, metabolic doctors believe, is during fasting. Dr. Jack Goldstein writes in *Triumph Over Disease by Fasting,* "The body in the fasting state is resting, and the use of exercise may put an excessive strain on the heart and other organs, with life-threatening consequences."[19] Otherwise, any exercise that keeps the heart rate at approximately 144 to 156 beats per minute, which should allow normal conversation during exercise, can be considered safe. This limit is the one commonly applied to cardiac patients.[20] Metabolic doctors recommend that exercise be engaged in to a point of stimulation, rather than overt fatigue. Exhaustion is believed to be quite counter-productive.

Many common exercises are recommended, depending upon what is enjoyed. During the administration of a metabolic program, people are advised to learn to do the things they enjoy—the time spent engaging in a metabolic program is not intended to be time spent learning how to punish oneself with drudgery. Jogging, hiking, basketball, swimming, dancing, and a great many other forms of exercise are all considered helpful.

Very compatible with the relaxed, pleasant state of mind that is considered so important for people with cancer is walking or yoga. Cancer research Dr. George Berkley believes walking is better for the physical and mental needs of cancer patients than are more difficult exercises. "A brisk daily walk," he says, "along with other forms of natural and non-competitive physical activity, may do much to keep us healthy and cancer-free."[21] Luanne Rona, M.D., says, "Walking gets the circulation going, breathing is improved, and it is invigorating to a tired or weary mind."[22]

Yoga is physically invigorating, easy to do even if one's energy level is reduced, can be done indoors or outdoors, alone or with others, and is mentally relaxing. A study performed at the Medical Institute of Benares at Hindu University in India showed that a program of yoga and meditation yielded substantial relief from several stress diseases, including ulcers, insomnia and hypertension.[23]

Muscular exertion is considered helpful, even to cancer patients who are bedridden, although this exercise may consist only of stretching, or lifting one's head or legs off the bed. As health returns, it is generally recommended that the exercise become more ambitious. Exercise abilities can be used to gauge returning health, but should not, of course, be forced to precede the natural healing rate.

For an ambulatory cancer patient, a daily program, say metabolic doctors, of light, pleasant exercise is recommended. The exercise can last up to one hour, if one's energy level permits. Exercising three times a week, say these doctors, should constitute a minimum exercise program.

Exercise is intended to lead to new activities, new friends, a new appreciation of the strength of the body, a respite from worry, and the pleasure of interacting vitally with the environment.

Rest

The importance of relaxation was established in the chapter, "The Emotional and Spiritual Aspects of Cancer."

Relaxation, though, is not always a state of mind that one can simply will oneself into. Often it takes a break from one's routine, and frequently extra sleep, in order to be able to fully relax. Resting, though, helps the body as well as the mind. It allows organs and glands a time for repair and regeneration, and rejuvenates the entire system.

It is reportedly characteristic of the cancer patient to fail to rest enough, particularly if the patient has a "go-getter" sympathetic-dominant metabolism, as many cancer patients seem to. It appears to be typical of the give-more-than-take attitude of the cancer patient to get up early, go to bed late, and fail to take a nap during the day. This type of behavior may be conducive to material success or to fulfilling all the expectations of one's family, but it is not considered conducive to overcoming cancer.

Harold H. Bloomfield, M.D., says in *Health and Happiness,* "The body needs to rest so that it can normalize the effects of stress and fatigue accumulated during the day. Rest is the basis of activity. The more profound the level of rest, the greater potential for dynamic, productive activity."[24] Dr. Bloomfield asks patients the following questions to determine if they are getting enough rest: (1) Do you take more than 20 minutes to fall asleep? (2) Do you wake up several times during the night to urinate? (3) Do you wake up during the night because of worries, hunger, dreams or discomfort? (3) Do thoughts frequently move too quickly through your mind? (4) Do you fail to wake up feeling refreshed? (5) Do you frequently have headaches, sore eyes, tired shoulders or lower back pain?[25]

Affirmative answers to these questions indicate possible lack of sufficient rest. Not enough sleep and relaxation causes restlessness, insomnia and physical discomfort.

People on a metabolic program may require additional rest, because of the extra stress involved in reversing their conditions. Naps during the day are considered to be very helpful, especially if taken after meals. Extra rest is also considered valuable in that it can force the patient into confronting the feeling of not being worthy of a respite from work or helping others. Sleep, which Shakespeare called the "chief nourisher in life's feast," is a very self-oriented activity. Engaging in it as much as one wants can help a patient to realize that his or her emotional and physical needs are important.

Smoking

All people with cancer are advised to stop smoking, even if they do not have obvious lung problems. Smoking decimates enzymes, leeches vitamins A and C from the bloodstream, overstimulates the nervous system, toxifies the entire system, decreases oxygen absorption, and harms the appetite. The cancer patient, say metabolic doctors, cannot afford any of these effects, let alone all of them simultaneously.

Metabolic doctors believe that smoking is one of the single most harmful health habits that any cancer patient can fall prey to. It is considered as harmful as eating junk food or being exposed to highly toxic industrial chemicals.

Nine out of ten smokers would like to quit. However, 39 percent of all men and 29 percent of all women now smoke, and percentages of the population that smoke decline only slightly from year to year.[26] In the group of five million Americans who smoke, there are definite social, economic and racial patterns. For example, one third of the population living with a spouse smoke, while half of those who are divorced smoke.[27] Nonwhites are more likely to smoke than whites by a 55 percent to 38 percent ratio. Men with college educations and high incomes are less likely to smoke than those with lesser education and income.[28]

Tobacco smoke contains thousands of components, many of which cause disease.[29] Especially harmful are tar, nicotine, carbon monoxide and the millions of solid particles that are drawn into the lungs, where most remain.[30] Nicotine is the agent that is most physically addictive.[31] Poisonous carbon monoxide, however, while not addictive, composes one to five percent of all cigarette smoke.[32]

Cigarette smoking alone is responsible for about 325,000 deaths each year, of the approximately two billion people who annually die in America. Cigarettes, then, account for about one death in every six. Cigarettes kill people by destroying the function of their hearts, blood vessels and lungs. About 90 percent of all lung cancers, the greatest killer of all cancers, are directly related to cigarettes. Besides lung cancer, smoking contributes to cancers of the larynx, pharynx, oral cavity, esophagus, pancreas and bladder.[33]

The risk of developing lung cancer is ten times greater for smokers than non-smokers. Cigarette smoking, when combined with certain occupations, chiefly those associated with gaseous or floating particulate pollution, is especially deadly. For example, asbestos workers who smoke have 92 times as much chance of contracting cancer as asbestos workers who don't smoke.[34]

Smoking is also the primary cause of chronic bronchitis and emphysema. Smokers have more frequent minor lung ailments than non-smokers, are subject to longer convalescence following illness or injury, and are more likely to develop post-operative infections.[35]

Return of health begins almost immediately after a person stops smoking. Within the first 12 hours after smoking is stopped, there is a rapid decline in the carbon monoxide level in the blood. Symptoms of cough, sputum production and shortness of breath improve within the first two weeks of non-smoking. After ten years of non-smoking, smokers' disease risks are equal to those of non-smokers.[36]

Though most people would like to stop smoking, the majority are unable to. This addiction appears to be related only partially to withdrawal symptoms caused by lack of nicotine. These physical symptoms, though they may cause discomfort, are not long in duration. Of more consequence may be remembering the sedative effects of nicotine use, which triggers desire.[37]

It is difficult for a smoker who is not sick to stop smoking, because he or she must relinquish immediate gratification for future benefit. Because nicotine takes only seven seconds after it's inhaled to reach the brain, and because the average smoker may receive as many as 70,000 of these immediately gratifying experiences of inhalation per year, smoking is unmatched by any other drug or habit as a source of immediate, frequent gratification.[38] These individual experiences are used by smokers to relieve anger, tension and boredom, to serve as a temporary escape, to provide physical relief from withdrawal symptoms, to provide mental stimulation, and to provide physical pleasure.[39] Balanced against these frequent and varied short-term benefits, the long-term drawbacks of smoking may seem insignificant to a healthy smoker. For a person with cancer, however, the benefits of stopping smoking are much more immediate.

Cessation of smoking is usually successful only when the smoker is actively involved in a non-smoking maintenance program. When maintenance is not a part of the program, about two-thirds of all people return to smoking after three months, and a long-term success rate of only 20 percent to 30 percent is achieved.[40]

Social-oriented stop-smoking programs seem to be among the most effective means to stop the habit, especially programs with a maintenance program that includes positive reinforcement with phone calls, letters, recorded messages, literature, visits with a therapist or group meetings.

Other forms of stop-smoking techniques include drug therapy, aversion therapy, fear arousal techniques, hypnosis and acupuncture.[41]

Drug therapies, generally involving tranquilizers, do not seem to be particularly effective. Aversion therapies, especially ones in which smokers are forced to smoke until they become ill from the tobacco, seem to have a relatively high initial success rate that quickly erodes. Fear arousal does not seem to work at all; actually it can have the opposite of the intended effect, causing an increase in smoking as a response to the stress of fear. Hypnosis and acupuncture, like aversion therapy, gain only short-term responses.[42]

Considering the positive aspects of non-smoking, and being supported by friends, seem to be the only effective ways to stop smoking. Once a smoker quits, many forces will be influencing him or her to begin again. A frequent reminder of non-smoking's benefits, and encouragement from others, are the strongest counters against these forces.[43]

Following are programs that may help people to stop smoking:

1. Smoke Enders
   3708 Mt. Diablo Blvd.
   Lafayette, CA 94549
   (800) 227-2334 / (800) 642-4772 in California

2. Seventh Day Adventist
   North American Health Services
   6840 Eastern Avenue, N.W.
   Washington, D.C. 20012
   (202) 723-0800
   Cost: Free - $25

3. Freedom from Smoking in 20 Days
   American Lung Association
   1740 Broadway
   New York, NY 10019
   Cost: $5

Two Anti-Cancer Lifestyles

Living an anti-cancer lifestyle may be a challenge to a person who has formerly led a carcinogenic lifestyle. But a healthy lifestyle is not an unpleasant one. It is, rather, one of growth, learning, pleasure and vitality. As a rule, people who adopt lifestyle changes as part of a metabolic program rarely return to most of the negative habits that composed their former, unhealthful lifestyles. They generally desire to avoid the lack of energy, shortage of mental sharpness, and emotional instability that are virtually wedded to unhealthy living.

Following are samples of typical days of recovering cancer patients. The first is that of Eydie Mae, as described in *How I Conquered Cancer Naturally.*

six a.m.: arise, cut and grind wheatgrass, take wheatgrass enema, then wheatgrass implant.

seven a.m.: exercise class, with stretching, yoga and relaxing.

eight a.m.: breakfast, followed by preparing juice for the day.

nine a.m.: attend lectures on health and participate in other intellectually stimulating activities.

eleven a.m.: wheatgrass implant, and drinking juices.

noon: lunch.

one p.m.: nap, followed by light exercise.

two-thirty p.m.: bake bread or prepare food.

three-thirty p.m.: coffee enema, or possibly colonic.

four-thirty p.m.: detoxification procedure, such as sauna or herbal bath.

six p.m.: dinner.

seven p.m.: drinking juices, relaxing, talking.

ten p.m.: bedtime.[44]

Dore Deverell, in *How I Healed My Cancer Holistically,* describes her participation in a metabolic program. Here is her schedule:

8:00 a.m.: drink juice.

8:30 a.m.: breakfast.

9:30 a.m.: coffee enema.

10:30 a.m.: drink juice diluted with water.

11:00 a.m.: swim at health club, or sun bathe or take sauna.

Noon: lunch.

1:00 p.m.: nap or short walk.

2:00 p.m.: meditation.

2:30 p.m.: drink juice.

2:45 p.m.: engage in pleasant activity.

5:00 p.m.: light dinner.

6:00 p.m.: reading.

9:30 p.m.: hot bath.

10:30 p.m.: bedtime[45]

As health returns, the schedule is gradually modified to include a normal, productive output of work and helping others.

These routines, obviously, are dissimilar to the standard American regimen of: gulp-your-breakfast, work-until-you-drop, belt-down-beer, and fall-asleep-watching-T.V. They are, though, hardly unpleasant, and can become a reward in themselves. They can also, according to metabolic physicians, help the body overcome cancer.

PART FOUR

The Changes In Your Life

We shall not cease from exploration
And the end of all our exploring
Will be to arrive where we started
And know the place for the first time.

—T. S. Elliot

CHAPTER SEVENTEEN

A Lifetime Change

Metabolic doctors say that the pervasive yearning in patients to disassociate themselves from their cancer is characterized by these patients' eagerness to believe that once the surgeon's skillfully-wielded scalpel has "gotten it all," the problem is over: kaput! A thing of the past! The "doctor's-gotten-it-all" belief is part of most people's externalization of the disease. People want desperately to believe that cancer comes from outside of them, rather than that it is a problem woven into the fabric of their lives. They are therefore quick to embrace the notion that once they have undergone medical therapy, the "invading" cancer has been driven for all eternity from their bodies.

This may be a comforting belief to bed down with, but it is a belief not likely to save one's life. In fact, say metabolic doctors, it is a myth, a myth that can kill.

Cancer, these doctors say, is a lifetime problem. It is a lifelong problem for those who never contract it, and substantially more of a lifelong problem for those who do contract it. A person who has never had a malignant tumor may one day play host to one, and a person who has had a malignancy is even more of a prime candidate for future cancer.

Cancer, as has been shown in this book, is not just one or more tumors—cancer is a condition. It is the result of the sum of one's diet, genetic structure, habits, living conditions, mind, structural makeup and spirit. Any number of factors can lead to the formation of cancer. If one creates within oneself a condition conducive to malignancy, then one will in all likelihood contract cancer. This may happen, of course, at any time, including the years following recovery from a malignancy.

In fact, recovered cancer patients are quite often the most vulnerable of all people to a bout with the disease. If they have suffered permanent damage to major organs or glands during the disease, if they received radiotherapy or chemotherapy during thier illness, if they failed to fully correct the lifestyle mistakes that led to their initial cancer or if their bodies still retain cells mutated by past exposure to chemicals or genetic heritage, they are spotlighted targets for further malignancy.

It is therefore important for all cancer patients, say metabolic doctors, to continue a modified version of their metabolic program throughout their lives. It is also highly advisable, they say, for people who have never had a diagnosable malignancy to engage in a modified metabolic program, as a cancer-preventive measure.

Adherence to a lifelong program does not indicate capitulation to paranoid cancer-phobia. A program has many immediate rewards. It is, say metabolic physicians, as effective at preventing minor ills, such as the flu or colds, as it is in preventing degenerative diseases, such as cancer and heart disease. It is also considered an excellent energy-booster and mood-stabilizer. People on long-term, modified metabolic programs, which are nothing more, and nothing less, than prudent health-stimulation programs, are thought by metabolic doctors to be among the most vital and emotionally balanced people one could imagine. Most recovered cancer patients reportedly tell metabolic doctors that they wouldn't return to their former cancer-causing lifestyles even if you paid them to do so. These people say they simply feel too good on a metabolic program to want to abandon it.

The Myth of the Five-Year "Cure"

One of the most entrenched fallacies in the field of cancer therapy is that if one is alive five years after initial therapy, one is cured. Five-year survival is the most common definition of a cancer cure. This spurious index of health is one of the prime inflators of cure rate figures obtained by the common, invasive therapies.

Lucien Israel, M.D., director of a French hospital and a consultant to the National Cancer Institute, deflates this fallacy in *Conquering Cancer.* "The fact that a patient survives for five years after an operation does not imply that he is cured," says Dr. Israel. "Precise statistics published by a few centers show that, because of metastases, mortality from cancer persists beyond ten years, and sometimes beyond fifteen years."[1]

Dr. Israel points out that the drop in mortality that occurs after five years is not a per-capita drop, but one based on total numbers of the patient population. "The number of recurrences drops after five years only because the total number of survivors has dropped significantly by then and continues to do so," he says. "In reality, the curves show that between one month and ten years, the rate of death remains constant."[2]

Dr. Israel continues: "Only a short while ago, patients with Hodgkins disease who had lived beyond fifteen years were considered cured. But recent studies have raised disturbing doubts: it seems that when autopsies were performed on certain of these patients after accidental death, they were found to have harbored perfectly identifiable uncured lesions. . . .[3]

"At present, there is no way of being absolutely certain that an individual case of cancer is cured. While it is true that the chances of cure increase with the passage of time, we must admit, if we are scrupulous, that 'cure' can be defined only statistically. . . . Fixing a five-year limit for purposes of evaluation is convenient, but it leads the medical profession to overestimate the percentages of cure, and hence to underestimate the possible importance of postoperative treatment in a total strategy for improving results."[4]

Dr. Israel indicates that about half of all cancer deaths occur between the fifth and tenth year after surgery, as was pointed out in the chapter on the positive and negative aspects of chemotherapy, surgery and radiation. With chemotherapy, surgery and radiation, survival with kidney cancer drops from 30 percent to 5 percent between the fifth and tenth years. With stomach cancer, survival drops from 25 percent to 10 percent during those years. In breast cancer, with lymphatic involvement, it drops from 50 percent to 25 percent.[5] With other cancers, a similar pattern exists during the fith to tenth year, and beyond.

The message to cancer patients is clear: just because you have no clinical evidence of tumors, you are not "out of the woods." Breathing a long sigh of relief after five years of absence of symptoms, and then returning to the beer, cigarette and Mighty Burger you were enjoying before the disease, can be, quite literally, a fatal mistake.

Carcinogenic Cures

Assuming that the cancer threat is over as soon as no tumors are obviously present is especially risky if the person with cancer has undergone chemotherapy or radiation: Both of these therapies often cause future malignancies. These treatments are directly carcinogenic—they cause genetic disturbances within the chromosomal network of the cell. They also inhibit the circulatory and lymphatic systems' immune functions, allowing future cancers to develop. These therapies can also, as can surgery, impair the function of organs and glands that are considered secondarily associated with immunity to cancer, such as the liver and pancreas. All of these negative factors can occur simultaneously. Because of these factors, patients who have undergone combined chemotherapy and radiation treatments experience an astounding twenty-five times the normal rate of cancer, as reported by Maugh and Marx in *The Science Report on Cancer Research.*[6] As science investigator Ralph W. Moss points out, "a person who is 'cured' of cancer by these drastic means (chemotherapy and radiation), may find himself struggling with a new drug-induced tumor a few years later."[7]

Probably the most pronounced cancer-promoting effects of these therapies are their direct carcinogenic attributes. It was first proven in 1902 that radiation can cause cancer; in that year a German doctor noticed that a tumor had developed on a patient at the exact site that had been repeatedly exposed to x-ray.[8] By 1906 it was known that radiation caused leukemia.[9] It is ironic that most early radiation-induced cancer deaths were those of the doctors who used x-ray for diagnosis and radiotherapy as a cancer treatment. One radiation-caused death was that of Marie Curie, the pioneer in the field of radiation.[10]

Radiation, according to Dr. Israel, induces genetic mutations that can cause the cell to lose its "memory" to stop dividing.[11] This genetic disruption can also cause birth defects in future generations, if radiation is applied to the testicles, as it often is.[12] Radiation can cause immediate problems by burning tissues, but its damage can also lie dormant for many years. Dr. Israel writes, "A few years ago it was learned that irradiation of the thyroid region during childhood is dangerous and, in a not inconsiderable number of cases, induces cancers in the adult.[13]

"It may seem curious," he writes, "to use ionizing radiation to treat diseases that can also be caused precisely by ionizing radiation. . . . Weak doses of radiation are mutagenic and can start the chain of phenomena that, over a period of several years, leads to cancer."[14]

Chemotherapy can also be directly carcinogenic, since it also disturbs genetic function. "Chemotherapy," writes Moss, "poisons many normal tissues . . . especially the rapidly dividing cells of the bone marrow, intestinal wall and hair follicles."[15]

National Cancer Institute co-founder Dean Burn, Ph.D., is quoted in *World Without Cancer* as saying, "Ironically, virtually all of the chemotherapeutic anti-cancer agents now approved by the Food and Drug Administration for use or testing in human cancer patients are . . . usually highly carcinogenic. . . . These now well established facts have been reported in numerous publications from the National Cancer Institute itself, as well as from throughout the United States and, indeed, the world."[16]

Therapeutic Assaults on the System

Metabolic doctors believe, of course, that cancer is the result of a complex chain of factors, rather than merely exposure to a chromosome-disrupting agent. At least as important as carcinogens in the formation of tumors, they think, is failure of the body's immune and reparative mechanisms to respond to the genetic insult. Chemotherapy, surgery and radiation, however, can have profoundly negative effects upon those systems of response.

Immune function is assaulted by chemotherapy and radiation. "Radiation," writes Dr. Israel, "can cause a severe and prolonged immune deficiency. This is true for radiation of the thymus, the organ in which the T-lymphocytes are processed, and hence for radiation of certain tumors of the lung, esophagus, and breast, among others. But it is also true of the radiation of large abdominal areas, which affect an extensive system of lymph nodes, bones, and blood vessels. The more the patient's immunological status deteriorates, the greater becomes the risk of both regional and distant metastases. From this point of view, we are beginning to suspect that radiotherapy is a two-edged sword. . . ."[17]

The assault of radiation on the immune system is especially hard to avoid, says Dr. Israel, when extensive areas of the body are exposed to radiation. "When a wide area is exposed to radiation, it is impossible to avoid irradiating large portions of the skeleton, and hence of bone marrow in which the different blood-cell lines are formed. The serious bone-marrow deficiency that would result if the entire body was irradiated is an insurmountable obstacle to such therapy, unless a bone-marrow graft is performed afterward, which is still an exceptional procedure."[18]

Chemotherapy can also be devastating to the immune system. Dr. Israel addresses this problem. "The lowering of immunity is only one aspect of the toxicity of chemotherapies. . . . Most of the cytostatics diminish immune response by blocking the proliferation of the leukocytes responsible for them. The result may be not only to facilitate the growth of the tumor but also, of course, to facilitate infections—microbial, viral or fungal—like those that are observed in patients with heart or kidney transplants. . . . The undeniable toxicity of chemotherapeutic agents is attributable to the fact that they are still almost totally nonselective, being picked up not by cancer cells in particularly but by all the tissues that proliferate fastest. These include the bone marrow (which manufactures leukocytes, red corpuscles, and platelets) . . . and certain endocrine glands."[19]

"The bone marrow," writes Moss, "is the foundation of the immune system. The use of chemotherapy is often accompanied by destruction of this immune system. . . ."[20]

Surgery can also harm immune function, if it disrupts or results in removal of important facets of the system, such as portions of the skeletal system, certain endocrine glands, or certain internal organs.

Suppression of the immune system is generally short-term. Even short-term suppression, though, can allow cancer to spread, then to lie dormant as it is held in check by the immune system. Long-term immune depression, however, may also be present in patients who undergo chemotherapy and radiation.

All of the invasive therapies also contribute to further cancer, according to metabolic doctors, by their general disruption of the body's overall metabolic processes. For example, removal of a large portion of the stomach, or damage to it by chemotherapy, would almost certainly hurt the body's ability to absorb the nutrients needed by the organs and glands most closely associated with immunity to cancer. Likewise, the assault on the liver caused by chemotherapy is not directly carcinogenic, but can exert severe cancer-promoting effects by limiting the body's ability to neutralize metabolic and chemical toxins. Even a factor like structural disturbance, caused by surgery, or emotional upset, caused by the pain or disfigurement of surgery, could tip the delicate balance of the metabolism towards a resurgence of malignancy.

The most common therapies for cancer, then, are indeed often dangerous to the patient who seeks long-term survival, rather than merely short-term improvement.

Cancer Causes Cancer

Invasive therapies are not the only factors that can lead to future cancer. Cancer itself exerts many of the same harmful effects that are associated with the invasive therapies. Cancerous masses secrete agents that depress immunity; tumors can cause poor function of the organs and glands of immunity by directly attacking them; tumors can harm many important organs needed for general health maintenance; and tumors can, of course, spread and then lie in a state of readiness, waiting for immune function to weaken.

A great many people with cancer suffer organ damage during the disease. Not only attack by tumors, but also extra organ and glandular exertion during the illness, can severely stress important organs and glands. It is the rare cancer patient, say metabolic doctors, whose liver, pancreas, thymus or kidneys are not greatly stressed during the formation and eradication of the disease.

Because of this organ and glandular stress during the disease, metabolic physicans try to rebuild optimum function of organs and glands during metabolic programs. The physicians temporarily substitute for and stimulate organs and glands during the recuperative phase of the disease, and also try to help rekindle these organs' and glands' proper functions. It is quite possible that certain organs and glands were not functioning properly before the disease, these doctors believe, since the disease was allowed to develop. These organs and glands are believed to be needed for future resistance to malignant growth. Stimulation and substitution can be carried on indefinitely, of course, but patients are advised to try to regain their own natural functions, so that external support and stimulation will not be necessary.

Cancer Patients Cause Cancer

Cancer is almost certainly a reflection of mistakes in living. Most of these mistakes can be corrected by the learning process of a metabolic program. The general tendency of people who have recovered from cancer is to continue their metabolic program after their health has returned, because the program boosts feelings of energy and well-being. Some people who have recovered from cancer, though, drift back into harmful habits similar or identical to the ones that led to the disease. These are often people who have tried throughout their illness to externalize the condition—to blame it on uncontrollable factors outside of themselves, or to credit their recovery to a particular vitamin or detoxification technique or physician.

People who resume their old, harmful habits, say metabolic doctors, are daring cancer to return. Everyone, to some degree, seems to return to harmful habits once their health returns. Some patients return to the eating of certain favorite desserts or to moderate social drinking. If this is done after they have regained their proper metabolic functions, and if it is done with restraint and intelligence, it generally doesn't seem to derail a person's health. If, on the other hand, a person's lifestyle begins to mirror the lifestyle that preceded the disease, problems may well be in the offing.

A person who has recovered from cancer must also remember that he or she is probably still carrying many mutated cells, similar to those that caused the original malignancy. Exposure to carcinogens five to thirty years earlier probably damaged more cells than just those involved in the former tumor growth. The person who has had cancer should accept the existence of these "time bombs," and take the proper steps to naturally deactivate them if they "explode."

Similarly, say metabolic doctors, a genetically-inherited weakness, quite possibly in an important anti-cancer organ, such as the liver or pancreas, may have been an important causal factor in the initial malignancy, and may be just as present in formation of possible future disease. A metabolic program should help the patient to overcome inherited weakness in a certain organ or gland, but this compensation may never be total.

People with cancer are, then, in all probability, people who began their programs with definite sets of bad habits, and possible organ or glandular weakness because of lifestyle abuse, genetic inheritance, or the ravages of the disease. They are people who may have been subject to the further insult of an invasive therapy. These combined factors have left them more vulnerable to cancer than the average person. The intelligent person with cancer will recognize this fact, say metabolic doctors, and act accordingly.

A Modified Metabolic Program

Engaging in a modified metabolic program throughout one's life is believed by metabolic doctors to be the proper response to the problem of being a person who has recovered from cancer. As health returns, people recovering from cancer are advised to gradually modify their programs. They are advised to eat a diet higher in protein, including meat and dairy products, and one less alkaline. They are allowed to eat fewer raw foods, drink less juice, and widen the variety of their food selection. Recovery brings with it occasional indulgences, such as moderate eating of sweets or higher-fat foods.

Fewer food supplements, including fewer enzymes, are recommended as the condition of malignancy is conquered.

Food supplementation often drops by as much as one-half after the first year, and half of that is frequently omitted after the second year, if recovery is proceeding smoothly. The need to take supplements at the peak of alkalinity, 3:30 a.m., diminishes as recovery occurs. Fewer digestive aids are recommended as the pancreas and liver become less involved with helping to break down tumor masses and toxins.

Structural, emotional and lifestyle changes are also scaled down as recovery takes place. Fewer visits to professionals—chiropractors, osteopaths, massage therapists, psychologists, etc.—are thought to be needed as health returns. Less stringent adherence to exercise, meditation and positive thinking programs can be afforded as full recovery occurs. As the person who is recovering feels stronger, he or she is allowed to abandon the 24-hour per day recuperative program that is often helpful for people just beginning a program. People who have begun to recover gradually begin to live a lifestyle closer to the one they lived before the disease. Less rest and relaxation are recommended and more work can be done.

Detoxification measures, say metabolic physicians, can be reduced after six months to a year on a metabolic program. Coffee enemas can be reduced to one a day, or possibly less, as health returns. Liver flushes can be done less often. Purges and fasts need not be engaged in regularly.

After disappearance of all signs of tumors, the person with cancer can, according to metabolic doctors, engage in a health-stimulating regime that does not require much time or effort. By the time symptoms have begun to diminish, the person who is recovering will probably have integrated the various components of the daily program, such as supplementation and detoxification, into his or her normal daily activities. Extra-time-consuming measures, such as regular daily exercise or meditation, are not considered absolutely necessary once recovery is well-established.

Most people who have recovered, though, appear to have come to enjoy most aspects of their programs by the time they have become healthy. They seem to enjoy taking time out of the day to focus on their own needs and goals, and they apparently enjoy the energy and emotional stability that a metabolic program helps to bring. Therefore, adherence to a modified program does not, for most people, seem a chore. A modified metabolic program constitutes, rather, for most people, a more positive, fulfilling, lifestyle than their old lifestyle. A modified program becomes, for most people, a daily reminder—actually, a daily celebration—of the fact that they are now cancer-free.

CHAPTER EIGHTEEN

Combining a Metabolic Program with the More Common Therapies

Cancer patients who choose to employ the most commonly used cancer therapies of surgery, radiation and chemotherapy are taking a difficult path back to health. These approaches are often painful, costly, disfiguring, and disruptive to future health. However, sometimes these approaches are needed. Frequently, they can save the patient's life.

Many patients undergo, during the course of their treatment, one of the more common approaches and the metabolic approach. Often, patients begin metabolic programs only after they have already exhausted the possibilities offered by the more common therapies. Less frequently, patients use metabolic programs to bolster their bodies for the upcoming ravages of proposed surgery, radiation or chemotherapy. Sometimes, both the metabolic and the more common approaches are engaged in simultaneously.

Metabolic physicians are convinced that metabolic programs will improve the success possibilities of the common therapies. They also believe, however, that sometimes these more common therapies can retard the recovery of a patient who is on a metabolic program. Nonetheless, invasive therapies are sometimes a necessity, most often during an acute, life-threatening crisis, when immediate tumor shrinkage is imperative.

Bolstering the More Common Therapies with a Metabolic Program

Surgery, chemotherapy and radiation, all destructive to the body's natural stability, virtually demand a companion health-stimulation program. Instead, in most cases, they are accompanied by bland and poorly nourishing hospital food, increased emotional stress, exposure to a variety of institution-borne viruses and bacteria, and a lack of fresh air and exercise. It is small wonder that many patients, unprotected by their unsupported defense mechanisms, die as a direct result of the highly stressful procedures that were designed to save them. This phenomenon is discussed at length in the chapter dealing with the positive and negative aspects of the common therapies. The assault by chemotherapy, surgery and radiation upon general health also exaggerates, by lowering the body's resistance, the uncomfortable side-effects of the procedures.

Surgery is one of the most stressful medical procedures performed, and it is generally the first-line of invasive defense proposed for cancer patients, whose bodies are already stressed by the malignancy and by the systemic weaknesses that are believed by metabolic doctors to have led to development of the malignancy. The harmful side-effects of surgery can be greatly reduced by participation in a metabolic program prior to and after surgery. Optimum nutrition, in particular, can help the patient withstand the rigors of surgery. Vitamins A, C and E, and the mineral zinc, are of particular benefit. Jonathan E. Rhoads, Chairman of the National Cancer Institute's National Cancer Advisory Board, advocated, in a statement to the N.C.I., increased nutritional support for patients undergoing surgery for cancer. He pointed out that even patients unable to eat could be given extra nutrients intravenously.[1]

Vitamin A is destroyed during heavily stressful situations, such as surgery. But it is needed by the skin and connective tissues to help heal surgical wounds. In the *American Journal of Surgery,* Dr. Merrill Chernov recommends that surgical patients be given up to 100,000 units of vitamin A after surgery.[2] Vitamin A is also helpful, as was demonstrated by Benjamin Cohen, M.D., of Massachusetts General Hospital, in fighting post-operative infection, which is one of the most frequent fatal post-surgical complications.[3] Dr. Cohen administered large amounts of vitamin A to one group of mice, then performed surgery upon that group and a group not given vitamin A. All of the group not given vitamin A died of infection, while the A-supported group uniformly developed and then overcame infection.[4]

Zinc, which is required for vitamin A synthesis, is also helpful for surgical patients. Ananda S. Prasad devotes an entire chapter in *Trace Elements in Human Health and Disease* to the benefits of zinc for surgical patients. He indicates that zinc is vital for "healing and repair," and demonstrates that many surgical patients are deficient in the mineral. Their deficiencies arise from "poor eating habits," . . . "inadequate intravenous feeding," . . . "the existence of the metabolic disturbances that initially created the need for surgery, and the fact that "anesthesia causes the blood levels of zinc to fall in the surgical patient."[5]

Use of vitamin C can improve the safety of surgery. In a British experiment, 30 of 63 surgery patients were daily given one gram of vitamin C before and after surgery. Of these 30 patients, none had serious problems with blood forming into clots, which is a serious post-surgical problem that can cause death. Of the 33 patients not given C, 60 percent had positive tests for clotting and 12 developed pulmonary clots.

Dr. Linus Pauling believes that vitamin C is essential during surgical and biopsy procedures to inhibit spread of tumors, which sometimes results from incision into the tumors.[6] Dr. Pauling says vitamin C can become severely depleted during surgery, and that it is "essential for the proper healing of wounds. . . ."[7] Without enough of it, he writes in *Vitamin C and Cancer,* "the patient can be plagued by serious and often fatal post-operative complications."[8] These complications include wound rupture, infection, pneumonia and cystitis.[9]

Vitamin E is also important for persons undergoing surgery. This vitamin has shown excellent ability to prevent clotting, to prevent scarring, and to enhance rapid healing of wounds. Alton Ochsner, M.D., formerly of Tulane University, says of vitamin E and surgery, "I am convinced that its use is extremely beneficial and at times life-saving."[10]

Other facets of a metabolic program, such as emotional

stress-reduction, exercise, and detoxification, can also help the surgical patient. These procedures create within him or her a favorable attitude, and a condition of health that helps the body resist infection and other complications.

Radiation and the Anti-Cancer Program

Several nutrients also lessen the negative side-effects of radiotherapy, while improving its tumor-killing abilities. "There is some evidence," writes Dr. Pauling, "dating back to the 1940s, to the effect that patients on relatively high vitamin C intake suffer fewer unpleasant side-effects during treatment by radiotherapy, and also that high vitamin C intake increases the therapeutic value of the high-energy radiation."[11]

The unpleasant side-effects of radiation—fatigue and nausea—are thought to be caused in part by the toxic stress upon the system created by tumor breakdown. Vitamin C, which is especially effective at neutralizing toxins, is thought to decrease the toxic side-effects of radiation by deactivating these metabolic toxins.[12]

Vitamin C improves the anti-cancer properties of radiation, Dr. Pauling says, by stimulating production of collagen, or connective tissue, which increases the ability of radiation to form tumor-encapsulating, scarlike connective tissue around tumors.

Vitamin C is depleted during radiation, depleted by malignancy, and depleted by emotional stress. Therefore, several grams per day, or more, is considered by most metabolic doctors to be a proper dose for a patient undergoing radiation.

Hoffer and Roy, in *Radiation Research,* note that Vitamin E can be effective in preventing damage to the red blood cells during radiation. In an experiment they cite, irradiated mice suffered complete destruction of some red blood cells, while irradiated mice that had been given supplemental vitamin E showed no red blood cell damage.

Vitamin A also appears to boost the anti-cancer effects of radiation. In an experiment at M.D. Anderson Hospital and Tumor Institute in Houston, application of vitamin A reduced by 25 percent the amount of radiation needed to control tumors in animals.[13]

Detoxification measures, such as coffee enemas, saunas and

liver flushes, are considered by metabolic doctors to also be helpful in removing toxic metabolic debris from the system. Metabolic doctors also maintain that the often debilitating fatigue caused by radiation can be countered to some degree with glandular extracts, with mild exercise, and with a careful diet high in nutrients. Positive-thinking exercises are also considered helpful during the long hours in bed that radiotherapy sometimes necessitates.

Chemotherapy and the Anti-Cancer Program

Chemotherapy, with its frequently intense nausea, can be one of the most physically and emotionally devastating of all cancer therapies. The procedure kills, as a reaction to toxicity, many of those who undergo it, as was shown in the chapter on chemotherapy, surgery and radiation. Chemotherapy can also figuratively kill one's will to live, because of its pronounced unpleasantness. A metabolic program, however, is said by metabolic doctors to reduce chemotherapy's side-effects, including the side effect of death.

"Patients taking high doses of vitamin C," writes Dr. Pauling, "are spared many of the unpleasant side-effects of cancer chemotherapy regimes." Chemotherapy, the administration of poisonous drugs, kills many of the body's cells, particularly the rapidly-reproducing ones, such as cancer cells, hair cells, and cells in the lining of the gastrointestinal tract. Its effect on the gastrointestinal tract, its general toxicity, and its killing of tumor cells, all combine to produce a reaction of often severe nausea and vomiting.

Chemotherapy reduces the ascorbate, or vitamin C, content in each of the immune system's lymphocytes, is quite likely to reduce normal nutritional intake of vitamin C, and is likely to deplete levels of vitamin C by causing emotional and biochemical upset.

Because of this depletion of vitamin C, and because of the increase of toxins that is almost certain to occur during chemotherapy, metabolic doctors generally recommend that all chemotherapy patients augment their vitamin C consumption by taking several grams, or more, per day. This extra vitamin C, which is a superb neutralizing agent of toxins, is believed to help inhibit nausea. It will also, as Dr. Pauling points out, "allow doses of chemotherapeutic drugs much larger than usual to be used to good effect."[14] Vitamin C also, he says, "potentiates the cell-killing effect of a number of cytotoxic drugs in common use. . . ."[15]

A patient described in the British medical journal *Lancet,* who had been given the nausea-causing drug levodopa, experienced almost total quelling of nausea following repeated applications of four daily grams of vitamin C.[16]

Vitamin E, another effective detoxifying vitamin, has shown ability to neutralize the toxins created by chemotherapy. It can help reduce nausea, and has also been shown to reduce the destructive effects of at least one chemotherapeutic agent, adriamycin, which causes heart damage. Use of vitamin E to prevent heart damage was reported in *Chemical And Engineering News.*[17]

In an N.C.I. experiment, one group of mice was given vitamin E prior to administration of a chemotherapeutic agent, while another group was given the agent without prior administration of E. Within one month, 85 percent of the mice not given E were dead, while only 15 percent of the mice given E died.[18]

Vitamin E is also helpful in reducing the side-effects of certain pain-killing drugs that are given to many cancer patients, according to Wilfrid Shute, M.D.[19]

Vitamin A can help some chemotherapeutic agents to penetrate malignant cells, says Lucien Israel, M.D. This can be quite helpful, because cancer cells are often able to resist penetration by the chemotherapeutic agent, causing the patient to suffer the negative effects without benefiting from the positive effects.[20]

As was previously stated, other detoxifying measures, particularly coffee enemas, are believed to help reduce the nausea caused by systemic toxicity and overload of the detoxifying organs, such as the liver and kidneys.

Because a metabolic program has extremely powerful anticancer properties of its own, say metabolic doctors, it will supplement invasive therapies with its own tumor-killing abilities. As Dr. Israel indicates, the most common therapies by themselves cannot be considered absolute anti-cancer measures, because it is virtually impossible to kill every single cancer cell in the body with these procedures. But these common therapies, he shows in *Conquering Cancer,* can give the body's immune mechanisms enough time to overcome the malignant cells that these therapies leave.[21] The stronger the immune system is, the more it will be able to help chemotherapy, surgery or radiology. And nothing is more strengthening to the immune system, in the opinion of metabolic doctors, than a metabolic program.

Metabolic Programs and Cachexia

Cachexia, or gradual wasting away due to inadequate nutrition, is a frequent cause of death amongst cancer patients. Patients undergoing chemotherapy and radiation are especially vulnerable to cachexia, because of the inhibition of appetite caused by these therapies (especially chemotherapy), because of the diversion of nutrients needed to compensate for the assault of the therapies, and because of the emotional stress that may accompany these therapies.

A special program of nutrition is believed by metabolic doctors to be the best possible remedy for cachexia. Often, hospitals recommend high-fat and high-sugar foods, such as milkshakes, to help cachexic cancer patients maintain adequate weight. Metabolic physicians find this a highly irresponsible remedy to cachexia in the cancer patient, given the metabolic factors associated with the disease. Cachexia, they believe, should be met with a program of vitamin, mineral and enzyme supplementation and a diet of whole foods. Supplements will aid assimilation of the food that is eaten, and supplements will reportedly decrease the side-effects of cancer and invasive therapies, which cause cachexia. A nutritional therapy program of fresh fruits and vegetables, lactic acid and milk products, nuts, whole grains, and juices, is believed to help solve weight loss, without overly stressing the weakened organs of digestion and elimination.

"Cachexia," Jonathan Rhoads, M.D., told the N.C.I., "can often be temporarily reversed by nutritional means. . . ."[22] Gio B. Gori, head of the N.C.I.'s Division of Causation and Prevention, recently reported a test in which cachexic cancer patients placed on a program of enhanced nutrition lived more than ten times longer than expected, sometimes up to five and six years.[23]

Cheraskin, Ringsdorf and Clark report a test at the Washington University School of Medicine, cited previously in this book, in which 64 cachexic, bedfast patients were rehabilitated for many months, some of them becoming fully active, when placed on a program of nutritional therapy.[24]

A metabolic program engaged in during treatment with chemotherapy or radiation is also believed by metabolic doctors to help prevent the cellular damage caused by these therapies, which may result in a future malignancy. Certain nutrients' powerful neutralizing effects on toxins, discussed at length in previous chapters, is thought to save many cancer patients from therapy-created recurrences.

Pain Lessened

A metabolic program is believed to also have a positive effect upon another factor that is frequently present in patients undergoing invasive cancer therapies, which is pain. Patients on a metabolic program very commonly report cessation of feelings of pain upon beginning a metabolic program, and report resumption of pain upon temporary cessation of a metabolic program. Much of the reason for this, of course, is because the program appears to stop new tumor growth, and therefore the invasion of nerves and tissues by malignant cells. However, a metabolic program is believed to also have a generally beneficial effect upon the nerves, due primarily to nerve-soothing nutrients, and to the calming effect on the nerves that detoxification appears to create. These effects are particularly helpful for patients suffering post-operative pain.

The B-complex of vitamins, as well as calcium and magnesium, have a soothing effect on irritated nerves, and can reduce pain considerably. Vitamin E increases oxygenation of tissues, which sometimes appears to lessen the effects of a locally painful condition. This phenomenon has been studied by the Shute Foundation of London, Canada.[25] Positive mental attitude and creative imagery, as shown by Dr. O. Carl Simonton and others, also can play an extremely helpful role in pain control. Certain herbs, such as valerian and hops, can reduce pain. Some structural adjustments also seem to relieve pain.

A metabolic program, then, can be of considerable benefit to those who seek help through invasive therapies. If all patients on chemotherapy, surgery or radition were on a concurrent program of immune-stimulation, nutritional and structural therapy, emotional counseling, and detoxification, these therapies would almost certainly, metabolic doctors contend, be more effective, and would be far less painful and destructive.

The Effect of the Common Therapies on a Metabolic Program

Often, metabolic doctors advise patients not to subject themselves to chemotherapy, surgery or radiation. The destruction of immunity, and the bombardment of the body with toxins, are the two most compelling reasons that prohibit most metabolic doctors from frequently recommending these procedures to a patient already on a metabolic program. Many metabolic doctors have seen cases in which patients were progressing well on a metabolic program, and then tried surgery, chemotherapy or radiation, to their ultimate detriment.

Another phenomenon that many metabolic doctors have observed is the tendency of patients who have had no prior invasive therapy to progress more quickly on a metabolic program than do those who come to metabolic physicians after having had chemotherapy, surgery or radiation. This may be because many of those who have undergone invasive therapy tend to be in a late stage of their disease. But many metabolic doctors believe that these patients' difficulties in responding are due more to the effects of their previous treatment than to the stage of their disease. They believe that previous treatment with chemotherapy and radiation is often as important a factor in dictating against recovery as is an advanced condition of the disease. The more chemotherapy or radiation patients have received, the less well they seem to respond to a metabolic program. A patient who has had a short course of four or five radiation or chemotherapy administrations is not considered to be severely handicapped in his or her ability to respond to a metabolic program. However, a patient who has undergone 40 to 60 sessions of chemotherapy or radiation will probably, according to many metabolic physicians, have a considerably more difficult time recovering than would a patient with no prior invasive therapy.

Balance and Common Sense

Often, however, metabolic doctors do recommend chemotherapy, surgery or radiation. Metabolic physicians, as a rule, tend not to be doctrinaire, dogmatic, or exclusive. They rarely oppose any approach that might help, merely because this approach may conflict with their general philosophies. And chemotherapy, surgery and radiation, quite obviously, can often be extremely helpful. Frequently, one of these common therapies makes all the difference in a patient's recovery. Tens of thousands of cancer patients are saved each year by chemotherapy, surgery and radiation.

Surgery or radiation are most often recommended by metabolic doctors in situations where tumor mass is threatening life. For example, a fast-growing brain tumor that is impinging upon vital neurological function may require a short course of irradiation. The blood-brain barrier makes brain tumors rather difficult to quickly shrink metabolically, and a temporary halting of growth, achieved through radiotherapy, might be helpful in allowing the immune system sufficient time to regroup its forces.

Occasionally, a quickly-spreading breast malignancy will respond more favorably to a metabolic program if a lumpectomy is performed. In other cases, tumor bulk may be so great that the lymphocytes are having great difficulty in penetrating the tumor; in these cases, surgical "de-bulking" may be indicated.

In some cases, a particularly virulent leukemia may be temporarily put into remission with chemotherapy, if the body's own immune response does not appear to be solving the problem. During the remission, say metabolic doctors, a metabolic program can once again help reassert the dominance of the immune system.

In all of these cases, it is advised that the metabolic program be continued during the surgery, chemotherapy or radiation. A metabolic program, say metabolic physicians, will probably diminish the side-effects of the therapy, will quite possibly improve the therapy's effects, and will help the body's immune system to reassert its power.

Used together, the more common therapies and metabolic therapy represent, in many cases, a patient's most effective help in the struggle to recover.

CHAPTER NINETEEN

A Program for Other Diseases

Metabolic programs, as the author has said repeatedly, are not the "magic bullets" for cancer. Cancer, in fact, is not even the specific "target" of metabolic rebalancing. Metabolic programs are designed to create optimum health within each patient's body. A state of optimum health, of course, rules out, by definition, a condition of cancer. It also rules out the existence of heart disease, arthritis, multiple sclerosis, asthma, allergies, diabetes, or any other chronic or degenerative condition. The goal of metabolic work, then, is much more ambitious than merely finding a method of reversing cancer. Metabolic physicians attempt to help people reverse, or at least stabilize, all degenerative and chronic conditions.

As was mentioned in the chapter, "The Metabolic Approach to Cancer," all high-quality metabolic programs, including those recommended by metabolic doctors who consult with Dr. W. D. Kelley, are based on the "non-specific" concept of health care. These "non-specific" programs are intended not for any *specific* disease, nor do they affect only one *specific* part of the body. They consist, rather, of programs that create optimum health, and thereby help the body to reverse *many* different diseases. And these programs work by improving the function of *many* parts of the body.

The thousands of patients who have consulted metabolic doctors over the past approximate decade have included patients with cardiovascular and cerebrovascular disease, diabetes, arthritis, multiple sclerosis, allergies, hypoglycemia, schizophrenia, alcoholism, deafness, obesity, chronic infection, drug addiction, depression, chronic fatigue, Crohn's disease, asthma, and a number of other relatively rare disorders. Metabolic physicians maintain that they have been approximately as successful in helping patients with these conditions as they have been in helping cancer patients. Some of these various conditions, they say, are more difficult than cancer to effect change in, such as multiple sclerosis and other nervous system disorders, but, according to many metabolic physicians, almost every pathology imaginable has, at various times, with various patients, responded well to a program of non-specific metabolic therapy.

Does this mean, then, that programs of non-specific metabolic therapy are the "magic bullets" for all manner of specific diseases? Of course not. For this to be true, metabolic doctors would have to have a "magic machine gun," and they have nothing of the kind. What they do have is access to a vast compilation of computerized information about health, metabolism and pathology, which they can draw upon to recommend individualized immune-stimulating and metabolism-enhancing procedures to patients. The superb recuperative mechanisms of the human body do the rest. These mechanisms deserve the credit for reversing this multitude of often baffling and complex ailments. If any "magic" healing agent exists, metabolic doctors maintain, it is to be found within one's own body.

The Non-Specific Concept

The non-specific concept revolves around two complementary axioms: (1) All diseases are caused by multiple factors, and require multiple-factor healing programs to reverse them; and (2) multiple-factor healing programs can cause simultaneous improvement in people with a variety of diseases.

The non-specific concept is one of the oldest principles in the history of medical science. It is the principle that formed the basis of Hippocrates' teachings, and was the primary theoretical model used by most physicians until the advent of mechanistic medicine. When medicine began to be mechanized and compartmentalized in the 1600s, the concept of specific causes and specific cures for specific diseases came into vogue.[1]

This theory of disease has predominated in medicine for the past 400 years, having heretofore withstood only occasional challenges from holistic-oriented physicians, organizations, and teachers. Only in the past decade has the doctrine of specificity been seriously criticized by a substantial, powerful minority of medical researchers and physicians.

René Dubos has advanced eloquent critiques of the theory that every disease has a specific, limited, cause and a specific, limited cure. Dr. Dubos, formerly of Rockefeller University, writes in *Ways of Health,* "The doctrine of specific etiology has thus constituted the most powerful single force in the development of medicine during the past century. But there is now increasing awareness that it fails to provide a complete account of most disease problems as they naturally occur, and especially of those which are most important in our communities today. In general, pathological states are the consequence of several determinant factors acting simultaneously; moreover, the manifestations of any given agent differ profoundly from one person to another. Causality and specificity are therefore much less apparent in clinical situations than they are in the laboratory. A few acute infectious diseases and nutritional deficiencies, of course, present clinical pictures so characteristic that they can be classified as true biological entities. What the patient experiences and what the physician observes, though, constitute generally a confusing variety of symptoms and lesions, rather than a well-defined entity. In most cases, a syndrome, such as anemia, cardiac insufficiency, gastric disturbance, and depression, is more in evidence than the unique pathological manifestations of a specific etiological agent.

"Furthermore, each noxious agent can express itself by a great variety of different pathological states. The phthisis studied by Laennec had little in common with the primary infection that is now the most common form of tuberculosis in our communities; yet both are caused by tubercle bacilli of the same virulence. Syphilitic aortitis, paresis, tabes, syphilitic roseola, a gumma, or a chancre, can all be caused by identical forms of treponema pallidum. A traumatic accident that would be fatal for an aged person might have but trivial consequences for a young adult. Thus the characteristics of a disease are determined more by the response of the organism as a whole than by the characteristics of the causative agent.

"To complicate matters still further, different agents can elicit similar reactions. Bacterial endocarditis in man and mastitis in cows used to be caused almost exclusively by streptococci. Now that streptococcal infections can be successfully treated with penicillin, other microbial species commonly become established in the lesions and thus give a new microbial etiology to these ancient diseases. Similarly, congestion and hypersecretion of the nasal mucous membranes can be caused by viral and bacterial infections; by inhalation of smoke, dust, allergens, or cold air; by migraine of vascular origin, by the administration of parasympatomimetic drugs; by sorrow and tears. . . .

"Since the body has only a limited range of reactions, its response to assaults of very different origin and nature is rather stereotyped. For example, an intestinal pathology which mimics that of typhoid fever . . . can be produced by injecting into the mesenteric nodes almost any irritating substance, even a rose thorn! . . . The General Adaptation Syndrome seems to constitute an irrefutable denial of the doctrine of specificity. . . .

"Simple cause-effect relationships involving only one variable are rarely sufficient to account for the natural phenomena of disease. The total environment and the *milieu interieur* constitute a multifactorial system, each component of which must be studied with regard not only to its own characteristics, but also to its effects on the other components of the system."[2]

Application of the Non-Specific Concept

All vitalistic, naturalistic healers throughout history have applied the non-specific concept to their patients. Hippocrates, Paracelsus, the early 20th century eclectic physicians, and the early homeopaths, all of whom were discussed in the chapter, "The Foundations of Metabolic Therapy," used the non-specific concept skillfully and effectively.

The concept is now being employed by a host of holistic health practitioners, including virtually all of those associated with Dr. W. D. Kelley. Throughout the country, holistic physicians are recommending multi-faceted healing regimes to their patients, and are achieving simultaneous remissions in wide varieties of pathologies.

Cheraskin, Ringsdorf and Clark, in *Diet and Disease,* discuss the application of similar nutritional therapies upon an assortment of diseases, including psychological disorders, cancer, coronary heart disease and atherosclerosis, and show how similar nutritional therapies can be employed to prevent infertility, congenital birth defects, mental retardation and obstetrical complications. Obviously, there is no "germ" common to both mental retardation and cancer, no "virus" that causes both atherosclerosis and birth defects.[3] Why then, in the literally hundreds of experiments cited by the authors, are these diverse maladies subject to vast improvement when they are treated with non-specific programs, involving nutrition, exercise, and absence of harmful chemicals? The answer, of course, lies in the body's inherent recuperative and protective mechanisms. If the body's organs, glands and systems are afforded the basic raw materials they require, and if each system is helped to relate properly to every other system, the body will be able to exert immense influence upon a wide variety of possible pathologies.

"Ecological observations have provided two essential conclusions regarding the nature of disease," write Cheraskin, Ringsdorf and Clark. "Namely, disease is the result of a constellation of factors and, second, it occurs in an endless series of gradations. The interplay of host factors and environmental challenges constitutes the only tenable basis for the etiology of health and disease."[4]

Another prominent researcher who has written about non-specific nutritional therapy for a wide variety of diseases is Dr. Roger Williams, who pioneered in establishing the importance of individualizing nutritional programs. Dr. Williams has shown that individualizing a nutritional program to suit the patient's own special metabolic needs is more important than individualizing a nutritional program to fit a particular disease. In *Nutrition Against Disease,* Dr. Williams discusses the use of individualized nutritional programs to help patients resist birth defects, obesity, dental disease, arthritis, senility, alcoholism, and cancer. Dr. Williams concurs with other holistic authorities in crediting the recuperative mechanisms of the body with accomplishing almost all healing. "No physician in his right mind," he says, "would claim that he had healed a broken bone simply because he set it."[5]

Two current, well-known healing programs that apply the non-specific concept to many different diseases are those of Max Gerson, M.D., and Luanne Rona, M.D. Both programs address the needs of patients suffering from a variety of degenerative and chronic illnesses, and both programs are aimed at establishing a state of high health and well-being in the patient.

In the preface to the book *Total Glow,* by Dr. Rona, a patient describes how he "personally met some people who have had gravely serious illness, including arthritis, heart disease, and terminal cancer, who have completely recovered after giving up drugs and other treatments and going on a sound nutritional health program. Others have found relief from asthma, diverticulosis, psoriasis, diseases of the liver, pancreas and prostrate, and headaches and backaches, all through the natural approach to life."[6]

Dr. Rona's program consists of nutritional therapy, exercise, and mind-oriented and detoxification procedures. "The most important element in this self-improvement program is the integration of the individual and the total approach to the entire physical and emotional unit," she writes.[7]

The late Dr. Gerson devised a program—still being widely administered under physicians working with Dr. Gerson's daughter, Charlotte Gerson Strauss—that combines primarily nutrition and detoxification. Dr. Gerson explains in *A Cancer Therapy* that "many diseases do not appear independently of each other. . . ."[8] "Chemical findings," he says, "bring us to the conclusion that several different types of pathological changes may occur as the consequence of a deep, general cause in the body, which we can subordinate under one leading idea—the law of totality, or the loss, or diminished degree, of 'healing power'. . . ."[9]

Clinically employing the non-specific concept is, in the final analysis, a fundamentally more sound approach to combatting disease, say metabolic doctors, than is the common practice of rather randomly and arbitrarily assigning different disease names to different combinations of symptoms, and then trying to eradicate each disease, or at least the major symptoms constituting it, with a single, specific pharmaceutical drug or surgical procedure. "The whole process of specialized symptomatic medicine," says Michael Smith, M.D., "is totally separate from the way life works."[10]

Case Histories of Diverse Diseases

Following are selected case histories chosen to illustrate the clinical effectiveness of the non-specific concept when applied to various, apparently unrelated pathologies. All of the following cases were patients of doctors who have attended seminars given by Dr. W. D. Kelley. All of the following patients were recommended programs of non-specific metabolic therapy.

C. F. Saskatchewan, Canada. Multiple Sclerosis.

C. F. was diagnosed in 1974 by her physician as having multiple sclerosis, a supposedly incurable degenerative nerve disease. She had previously had western equine encephalitis. Several specialists failed to slow the course of the disease, and she was confined to a wheelchair in 1974. After beginning a non-specific metabolic therapy program in 1976, she radically changed the various components of her lifestyle. In six months she noticed improvement in her muscle control. After 1½ years she became fully ambulatory, totally symptom-free, and in good health. She has been diagnosed by three specialists as having no evidence of the disease.[11]

M. I. Colorado. Infertility.

The patient, 35, had been trying to conceive for some time but had been unable to. A patient evaluation procedure administered by her physician revealed she had a severe lack of cellular protein. She began a metabolic program in 1979, and became pregnant within two months. The pregnancy was full-term and the baby was healthy. She had previously been eating what she considered a very healthy diet.[12]

B. C. Connecticut. Pulmonary Congestion.

The patient has wheezed badly since childhood, and had been unable to reverse the condition through any previous therapy. He had been eating wholesome food, but his diet was found to be unsuitable for his metabolism. A patient evaluation procedure indicated that he had deficiencies in several minerals and also had adrenal dysfunction. After three weeks on a metabolic program, he reported having more stamina than he had had for many years, and the wheezing completely abated.[13]

J. A. M. New Jersey.
Degenerative Collagen Vascular Disease.

The patient, in her mid-40s, had a 20-year history of a slowly progressing degenerative collagen vascular disease, which was causing increasingly severe pain and stiffness in her joints and back. She had extreme limitation of motion and required crutches for walking, in spite of frequent, repeated treatment with pharmaceutical drugs. After beginning a nonspecific metabolic program, designed to meet her individual needs, she responded dramatically. Her pain and stiffness gradually disappeared. Within two years, she was markedly improved, and continued to improve steadily after that.[14]

J. B. M. New Jersey. Asthma.

The patient had had asthma and low energy for several years prior to beginning a metabolic program. He had been taking cortisone pills for the condition, which were discontinued after his program began. His asthma abated quickly after he began his program, and did not return even during periods of heavy exercise. His energy level also improved, and he became more resistant to minor ills.[15]

B. D. Illinois. Deafness.

B. D., 48, became totally deaf in 1977, diagnosed at a Chicago hospital as having acute labyrinth edema. Specialists in Chicago and California told her that the condition was irreversible, after unsuccessfully flushing her blood and treating her with antihistamines. After one year on a metabolic program, hospital tests confirmed that her hearing had begun to return. It improved over the next several months. She still has hearing difficulty, but can verbally communicate quite well. After her program began, she also reported a rapid improvement in her feelings of strength and vitality.[16]

S. M. Wisconsin. Crohn's Disease.

S. M. had suffered from Crohn's disease, a supposedly incurable chronic inflammation of the small intestine, for six years, with symptoms of anemia, underweight, high fevers, diarrhea, depression, low blood pressure and stomach cramps. No medical treatment improved the condition, including application of steroids, antibiotics and tranquilizers. She began a metabolic program in 1977 and responded positively within three weeks, with no concurrent medical therapy. In two months, most of the symptoms were gone, and in six months almost all were gone. The disease has never returned.[17]

F. B. Arkansas. Hypoglycemia.

The patient was diagnosed as having hypoglycemia in 1972, showing symptoms of severe fluctuations in mood and energy. None of the diets or therapies recommended by doctors and nutritionists helped. In 1977 she began a non-specific program. A patient evaluation procedure indicated that she was dysfunctional in several glands, that she had severe allergies, and that dietary compensation alone was not sufficient to reverse her apparently interrelated allergic/hypoglycemic problems. After six months on a metabolic program, she was substantially improved. After one year, she had no remaining symptoms.[18]

Non-Specific Metabolic Therapy and Cancer

Cancer, say metabolic physicians, is promoted by many negative factors, all of which complement the harm of the others. Negative nutritional, structural, emotional and lifestyle factors combine, say these doctors, to overcome natural immune resistance. Sometimes cancer therapies that address only one or two of these causal factors are successful. However, the best guarantee against death by malignancy, according to metabolic physicians, is a full-scope program that simultaneously addresses all of the major components that have an impact upon health and disease. This form of therapy—non-specific metabolic therapy—will, it appears, help the body to solve a multitude of physical problems.

CHAPTER TWENTY

The Experiences of Twenty People

Following are twenty selected case histories of patients who recovered while using a metabolic program administered by a physician who uses the computer consultation services of Dr. W. D. Kelley. The case histories were selected on the basis of variety of disease, virulence of disease, and by having been diagnosed at least five years prior to the publication of this book. Five-year remission is one of the criterion used for determining cure from cancer. Another criterion is showing no signs or symptoms of cancer, which none of these twenty patients do at this time.

The fact that all of these twenty patients recovered is not meant to indicate that all patients on a metabolic program recover.

(1) A. R. Louisiana. Prostate cancer, metastasized to pelvis. Diagnosis: terminal.

A carpenter, A. R. began having difficulty urinating and experienced discomfort in his prostate region in 1975, culminating in total inability to urinate in October 1976. Doctors at his local hospital in Louisiana made an initial diagnosis of an enlarged prostate, and arrived at a diagnosis of prostate cancer within two weeks. Further clinical examination revealed a lesion in his left ureter. His physician placed him on a brief course of radiotherapy to the chest region in preparation for surgical removal for the prostate. Further testing revealed a malignancy in the pelvic area, so prostate surgery was not attempted. A diagnosis of terminal malignancy was reached, but an orchidectomy (castration) and application of female hormones were performed to extend his life expectancy. The patient became progressively weaker, drainage from the kidneys was impaired, and he was confined to the hospital for five weeks. The patient read about the metabolic approach to cancer and began a metabolic program. Within four weeks, the lesion on the left ureter was gone and normal kidney function returned. Blood tests, bone scans and physical examinations done seven months after beginning his metabolic program revealed no discernible malignancy. The patient's appetite improved, 20 pounds of lost weight returned, mental outlook improved, and muscular strength improved. The patient is now at the same level of physical strength as he was prior to the disease, and has no symptoms of cancer.

(2) B. J. F. Washington. Metastasized skin cancer.

After removal of numerous nonmalignant skin growths and a nonmalignant growth on her foot over several years time, the patient was diagnosed by biopsy as having skin cancer in 1971. The malignant growth was removed, causing scarring, but another on the chin returned, which caused pain. Her physician determined that the cancer had metastasized, and recommended chemotherapy and further surgery. The patient declined, unwilling to be further scarred by surgery. She read about the metabolic approach to cancer and began her program in 1972. She experienced several symptoms of healing crises over the next two years, but otherwise recovered normally. The physician who had diagnosed the metastasized malignancy determined in 1974 that she was cancer-free. She now works full-time, has had successful cosmetic surgery for her facial scars, and reports feeling very good.

(3) W. M., Sr. Florida.
Prostate cancer metastasized to rectum.

For several years prior to diagnosis of cancer, W. M. suffered from prostatitis, required frequent attention from his urologist, once had a benign nodule on his prostate, had an apparent kidney infection, and had pain in his rectal area. In 1971 he was operated on for prostate cancer. A year later cancer reappeared in his rectal area. Another operation was performed, but symptoms of cancer continued. A family member recommended he begin a metabolic program, which he did in 1974. After a year on the program, and after suffering symptoms associated with tumor elimination, clinical tests and x-rays determined no continuing malignancy. At age 67, the patient is now very active and has no signs of cancer.

(4) V. S. L. Pennsylvania.
Liver cancer, multiple metastases. Diagnosis: terminal.

The wife of a minister, Mrs. V. S. L. had eaten well and lived a healthy life, but in 1973, at age 58, she was diagnosed by exploratory surgery following abdominal discomfort as having inoperable liver carcinoma, with several metastases. Her surgeon told her that she was terminal, and had a very short time to live. She was told about the metabolic approach to cancer by a local doctor and started a program. She received a very brief course of chemotherapy but stopped it abruptly against her physician's advice. After only about a year on her metabolic program, she had fully recovered, and was diagnosed as being free of cancer at her local hospital. She remains free of malignancy eight years after initial diagnosis.

(5) K. M. Florida. Uterine cancer with multiple metastases. Diagnosis: terminal.

The patient began experiencing prolonged weakness and abdominal pain after the birth of her second child in November 1967. Various diagnoses, including psychosomatic illness and premature menopause, were made, prior to a diagnosis of uterine cancer arrived at by biopsy. She was unable to urinate, was bloated, was in pain, had difficulty breathing, and could not keep her balance. Her surgeon diagnosed her cancer as corionepithelioma and told her she was terminal. Her cancer had spread to her liver, lungs and kidneys, and pancreatic involvement was suspected. No therapy was proposed. Friends told her about a patient who had recovered from cancer on a metabolic program, so she began one. After carefully following an intensive program for one month, she returned to her physician. He expressed considerable surprise that she was still alive; her kidneys had stopped functioning and he had thought she would be unable to live longer than a few days. He encouraged her to remain on her program. She experienced several relatively severe healing reactions, but was pain-free within seven months. Her strength returned and she was eventually diagnosed as having no more malignancy.

(6) L. B. Arkansas. Uterine cancer.

Suspecting uterine problems, L. B. had a PAP smear in December of 1972, which indicated no problems. Two months later, however, doctors at a Rochester, Minnesota, hospital told her that her entire uterus was filled with malignant growth. She quickly became too fatigued to even walk, and lost 30 pounds. She underwent no invasive therapy. She heard about the metabolic approach from a physician and began a program. She recovered quickly and completely. She is now very active, in good health, and shows no evidence of malignancy.

(7) H. S. O. Florida.
Pancreatic cancer. Diagnosis: terminal.

In 1974 the patient began experiencing episodes of prolonged nausea, and discoloration of the urine and skin. One week of hospital testing revealed nothing, but surgery for possible gallbladder pathology revealed a large malignant lesion, occupying the head of the pancreas and extending downwards. Palpation indicated that the pancreas was firm, nodular and enlarged. There was also malignant growth on the left posterior portion of the pancreas. The tumor was inoperable. The patient was given approximately one to eight months to live. No medical therapy was suggested. The patient's wife was familiar with natural therapies for degenerative diseases and recommended he begin a metabolic program, which he did within a few weeks. Within two months, the patient was fully active, was running his business, and eventually recovered with few significant problems. He has remained free of malignancy, and has not missed a day of work in several years.

(7) J. R. M. Arizona. Testicular cancer
with multiple metastases. Diagnosis: terminal.

A 65-year-old chiropractor, J. R. M. was diagnosed by an oncologist as having cancer in his testicles in 1975, after clinical and laboratory tests and a bone scan. The testicles were removed and radiation and chemotherapy were begun. After three months of these treatments, which proved ineffective, the patient was advised that the cancer had metastasized to several abdominal sites, and that he was terminal and beyond the help of palliative medical therapy. After being told about the metabolic approach by a friend, he began a program in early 1977. By November of that year, he was able to begin seeing patients again. Twenty pounds of lost weight returned. He became free of malignancy and now reports being in extremely good health.

(9) T. C. M. Louisiana. Acute granulocytic leukemia.

In August 1976, following a long period of bleeding, irregular heartbeat, fever, and weakness, the patient was unable to overcome a massive infection. Acute granulocytic leukemia was diagnosed and doctors told the patient, age 62, that there was very little hope of recovery. Antibiotics were the only medical therapy recommended. The patient began a metabolic program while still in the hospital, against his doctors' advice, at the urging of his wife. A remission from the leukemia ensued, which was followed by total disappearance of all symptoms of cancer. Muscle tone, strength and mental outlook improved markedly, and the patient is now very active and free of all malignancy.

(10) F. Y. Iowa. Uterine cancer, metastasized to the bladder and other sites. Diagnosis: terminal.

The patient required surgical removal of benign cysts and lumps over 15 years time, beginning in 1955. Her resistance to minor ills and her energy level tended to diminish after surgeries. In 1971, complaining of abdominal discomfort and digestive problems, she was diagnosed through exploratory surgery as having a large tumor in her uterine area. The tumor had grown through her uterine wall and was attached to the right ovary. The uterus, fallopian tubes and ovaries were removed. The surgeon told her that all of her cancer had been removed. Over the next year she had continued feelings of ill health and discomfort, discoloration of skin, and problems with frequent urination. In November 1972, further tumors were removed from the bladder, but other abdominal tumors were inoperable. She was told she was terminal. She was placed on a chemotherapy program, and stayed alive for two years. The chemotherapy did not eradicate the malignant growth, however, and surgery was proposed. She declined further surgery and, at the urging of a cancer patient who had recovered on a metabolic program, began her own program in late 1974. She recovered gradually without further surgery or chemotherapy. In 1977, after an automobile accident and cessation of her program for several months, she developed what seemed to her to be, based on previous symptoms, abdominal tumors. Upon resumption of her program, the symptoms disappeared. She now has no further symptoms of cancer and reports feeling good and being very active.

(11) M. D. Iowa.
Breast cancer, multiple metastases. Diagnosis: terminal.

In 1968 M. L. had a colonic obstruction. In May 1971, she underwent surgical removal of an intraductal papilloma and fibrocystic disease from her left breast. She was suffering concurrently from hot flashes and irregular menses. In January 1973, the patient, having discovered a nodule in her left lower breast, consulted an internist, who found a malignant mass in the left upper breast. Diagnosis of cancer was confirmed by xerogram and biopsy. Two of 21 nodes examined were found to contain metastases, and the patient was told she was terminal. She began a metabolic program almost immediately, and recovered quite quickly. By July of 1973 a chest x-ray showed no evidence of malignancy. Since 1973 she has suffered from slight discomfort in the right upper quadrant and has had her gallbladder removed, but has shown no further signs of cancer and is very active.

(12) L. N. Ohio. Breast cancer.

In 1972 L. N., a registered nurse, was diagnosed as having a malignant mass in her chest. She refused surgery and radiation, and immediately began a metabolic program. After one year of strict adherence to the program, her tumor had detached from the tissue in her breast but was still present. After modifying her diet, the malignancy completely disappeared. She is now working again, regularly plays competitive sports, such as tennis, and reports feeling quite healthy and energetic.

(13) B. A. B. California. Bladder cancer.

The patient, 74, was diagnosed as having bladder cancer in 1975. Her physician told her that there were at least five tumors inside the bladder. The physician recommended surgery, but the patient resisted, so she was placed on a chemotherapy program. After her sixth chemotherapy treatment the physician told her that the drug therapy was not working; he insisted that she have the bladder surgically removed. The patient withdrew from the physician's care and began a metabolic program, which had been researched and recommended to her by her daughter. After two years on the program, examination at a Kaiser Permanente Hospital showed that only one tumor remained in her bladder. Within six months, further examination showed her to be free of any malignancy. She is now very healthy, takes care of her own apartment, drives a car, works three days a week, and is in good spirits.

(14) U. M. Montana. Metastasized bladder cancer.

In 1975 the patient noticed an increasing sense of fatigue, coupled with insomnia. In December 1976, he noticed blood in his urine; within a month his urine was heavily saturated with blood. He suffered from discomfort while urinating, extreme fatigue, and frequent urination. On December 30, 1975, visual inspection of the bladder through surgery in a southern California hospital revealed a large tumor on the floor of the bladder with frond-like fingers extending upwards. The tumor had penetrated the bladder wall, and there were numerous small tumors scattered throughout the area, all malignant. Part of the large tumor was removed during the operation. The surgeon told the patient there was no further metastases of the bladder cancer. The patient chose to transfer directly to the M.D. Anderson Tumor Institute in Houston, where it was revealed that the cancer had spread to the lymphatic system. He began radiotherapy in January 1976, which was to be followed by removal of the bladder. Five days after the radiation treatment had begun, the patient was contacted by a nephew who was familiar with the metabolic approach to cancer. The nephew suggested the patient begin a program and forego the prescribed 20 remaining radiation treatments and surgery. Within two days, the patient stopped his radiotherapy and began a metabolic program, having studied materials sent by his nephew. The patient began almost immediately to notice small improvements, but developed a bladder infection. The bladder infection abated within two weeks, and the patient began to feel substantially better. Throughout the spring of 1977, the patient was weak and slept much of the time, but continued to feel better. After several relatively mild healing crises, the patient gradually stopped having any symptoms of cancer. His fatigue ceased, his mental attitude improved, and all urinary problems and pain ceased. Recent urinalysis failed to detect any signs of malignancy. The patient is now feeling good and is fully active.

(15) M. H. Minnesota. Colon cancer, metastasized to the liver. Diagnosis: terminal.

In the fall of 1974, M. H. began to be abnormally tired at the end of the day. A February 1975 complete physical, though, revealed no pathologies. She developed discomfort in her lower abdomen and was given a barium enema, which resulted in a diagnosis of colon cancer. She received a colostomy. After the surgery, inoperable cancer of the liver was discovered, after which she was pronounced terminal. Her surgeon recommended chemotherapy as a possible life-extending measure. She had heard about the metabolic approach to cancer and explained it to her surgeon. He was not supportive of the approach. Nonetheless, she began a program in March 1975. She changed her diet and lifestyle drastically, and recovered steadily. Within eight months her condition was significantly improved, and by April 1978, there were no remaining symptoms or clinical indications of malignancy. The patient now leads an active life.

(16) S. S. California. Hodgkin's disease. Diagnosis: terminal.

In 1971 the patient was told that he had an advanced, terminal case of Hodgkin's disease, a cancer of the lymphatic system. He had had symptoms of the disease for a relatively long period of time prior to consulting a physician. He was placed on a chemotherapy program, but felt that this therapy would be painful and hopeless. Therefore, he discontinued the therapy after the first few treatments. Doctors advised him to have his spleen removed, but told him he could only live for about ten months. Only 21 years old, the patient was told by a friend about the metabolic approach to cancer, and began his in 1971. After three months on a program, his lymphatic glands began to swell. This was the first of several healing crises. Within one month, the swelling went away and the patient felt markedly better. He followed a rigorous program and improved steadily. In 1974 he returned to the physician who had diagnosed his condition, and was found to be free of malignancy. In 1977 he underwent testing at Stanford Medical Center in California, and was found to be in excellent health. He is still quite healthy and is very active.

(17) E. H. California. Uterine cancer.

In 1970 E. H., 22, developed a fast-growing tumor in her uterus, even though she had lived a relatively healthy life and had eaten prudently. She did not follow the recommendation for surgery made by her family doctor, but, upon the advice of her mother, who was knowledgeable about natural healing modalities, began a metabolic program. She had several healing crises, and suffered from several long bouts of depression, but within two years her malignancy was in total remission. She is still quite healthy and shows no signs of cancer.

(18) P. B. Arizona. Lung cancer, metastasized to the esophagus. Diagnosis: terminal.

P. B., a chemical compounder living in Akron, Ohio, had surgery in 1975 after he had experienced pulmonary problems. His surgeon discovered malignancy throughout the lungs and a tumor wrapped around the esophagus. Part of the esophageal cancer was removed, but the lung cancer was inoperable. He was given nine months to live, if he participated in a radiotherapy program. He did 24 radiation treatments over one month, but the treatments were not eradicating the masses of tumors. He saw some written material on the metabolic approach to cancer and discussed the possibility of going on a program with his physician, who advised against it. In August 1975, he began a metabolic program and adhered to it faithfully. He moved away from the polluted air of Akron to an area of clean air, quit working as a chemical compounder—a profession associated with extremely high incidence of cancer—and followed the diet, supplementation and detoxification facets of the program carefully. Within 18 months, he was considered improved, and testing done in 1978 revealed that no further malignancy existed. He is still healthy and now works full-time.

(19) E. P. California. Uterine cancer with multiple metastases. Diagnosis: terminal.

In the spring of 1975, a malignant tumor was removed from the uterus of E. P., who was placed on a program of chemotherapy and radiation. However, a malignancy developed in her breast, and she was told that she would not recover. Her doctors recommended she have a mastectomy. She refused to have this surgery, refused further chemotherapy and radiation and began a metabolic program, having seen written material on the metabolic approach. After radically altering her diet, and following the other facets of her program, she began to recover. She experienced several healing crises. Further examination by the physician who diagnosed her condition showed that the cancer had gone into full remission. She remains healthy and active.

(20) K. M. Arkansas. Pancreatic cancer. Diagnosis: terminal.

K. L. was 15 when she was diagnosed in 1976 by an internist as having an advanced pancreatic cancer. He recommended she begin a chemotherapy program to extend her life. Her mother had already recovered from breast cancer on a metabolic program, so K. L. was advised by her mother to begin a metabolic program immediately. She received no surgery, radiation or chemotherapy. She was very weak at first, and had difficulty digesting food and remaining ambulatory. After one year, however, most of her symptoms had abated. Approximately 18 months after she began her program, her internist tested her clinically and found no evidence of malignancy. Now 20, she is very healthy, works in the health field, and goes to college.

EPILOGUE

What a Program Promises

Cameron Stauth is reminded of the first time he met Dr. William Donald Kelley: The doctor—leery of yet another sensation-sniffing reporter trying ever so hard to top all previous bests in the national arena of big-time Show and Tell. The journalist—loathe to waste a weekend on yet another Great American Doctor, that unique sub-species of the beast "Egotistus Bombastus," a breed whose blimp-sized egos croon constantly in their ears that *they alone* represent the world's salvation.

The doctor kicks off the interview, conducted in the only restaurant in the doctor's little town, by blurting, "If we don't change the whole course of medicine, we won't have accomplished a thing!" A headline materializes in the reporter's mind: "Doc Declares War on Medicine!! Establishment Vows Revenge!!" The reporter is thinking that, with any luck, he will soon be able to goad the good doctor into one or two more outrageous statements, and maybe even milk a little defamation of character out of him, whereupon the reporter will be able to wrap up his story and hit the ski slopes without even spending another buck-fifty on Memorex.

"I have heard," mumbles the reporter, *sotto voce,* leaning close in his best just-between-you-and-me-pose, "that you give seminars in which you tell medical doctors how they can cure cancer, even though you're a dentist rather than an M.D."

"I teach them some things I've learned about health," he says. "And then they teach their patients. If anyone does any curing, it's the patients who cure themselves."

"That may be an accurate description of the process, thinks the reporter, but it's *no headline.*

Well, whether it's the doctors you teach or the patients themselves who are doing the curing, isn't it true that an unusually high percentage of these patients are recovering?"

"I wouldn't even know what the percentage is," says Dr. Kelley. "I never discuss that with doctors, and I advise them not to discuss it with patients. I think it's arrogant of a doctor to offer a patient such-and-such a chance of surviving if they use a particular approach. So much of a patient's chances for survival depend on the patient's willingness to *work* for survival. I recommend to doctors that they offer patients just one thing, and that they offer each patient an equal amount of it." The doctor stops talking.

"Well," says the journalist, "what is it?"

"What would you guess it is?"

A couple of dirty-coveralled farmers stop by the table to talk to the doctor, giving the journalist a chance to ruminate. Through his mind run these thoughts: If this is a sub-species of Egotistus Bombastus known as the "Big-Hearted Guru Type," he'll say, "it's love." If it's a "Mr. Wizard Egotistus," he'll say, "the finest, state-of-the-art health care now available anywhere on earth." If this is a "Dr. Schweitzer Was a Rip-Off Artist Compared to Me" type of hyper-humanitarian, he'll say "treatment whether they can pay for it or not." But as the journalist thinks, he can clearly see that the doctor is actually talking to these . . . *ungrammatical* . . . people in coveralls, and is not condescending to them. Strange. The farmers leave.

"Figure it out?"

"Hope?"

"You're a smart kid. Let's go over to the Foundation."

The "Foundation," or Kelley Foundation, it turns out, is a little bit short on alabaster pillars, spacious grounds and white-coated lab assistants running around with styrofoam cups of coffee. The Foundation consists of a little house that could have been picked up, at that point in time, which was just before the mid-1970s real estate boom, for the price of a decent used Chrysler. The doctor, it seems, has sunk most of the liquid assets he's accrued over the last ten years into a series of computers that would make Harvard's physics department salivate with jealousy. The rest of his savings has gone to the phone company, which has kept him connected with about a hundred doctors around the country who have been attending his seminars and using his computer consultation services.

More impressive than the hardware, though, is a middle-aged, Enid, Oklahoma woman in the reception area, a woman who has recovered from a verifiable case of metastasized liver cancer that had once been so widely spread that it had filled virtually her entire abdominal cavity.

The woman has come, with her second-cousin, to visit the man who daily consulted with her doctor during the grim days of her disease. Her cousin has cancer.

Her cousin has insisted on coming here so that he can meet this man, observe his work, and survey his surroundings.

The cousin is a tired-looking old man, a man with a chalky face, a man with a foot in the grave. He seems dubious, and allows that, well, maybe her case did respond, but he'd been told that no drug, no surgery, no doctor, no machine, *no agent known to medicine,* could stop his cancer.

The journalist interrupts them to intimate that this Dr. Kelley must, indeed, be some sort of medical genius to have helped the woman's doctor cure her of cancer.

"Hey," she booms, suddenly alarmed, as if the journalist has just tried to snatch her purse, "don't get me wrong—Dr. Kelley's number one in my book, and my doc back home is number two. But *I'm* the dog that did this trick! *I am!*" She slaps her sides in triumph.

When she says this, something clicks in her cousin's eyes. Something that had not been in the old man's eyes five seconds before is—click!—there now. He sits up straight.

Dr. Kelley comes out to the reception area to invite the old man into his private office. The doctor does not have a receptionist. "Want to come back now?" He stands close, a hand ready to help the man up. The old man sees the hand. He doesn't take it.

He stands up. Alone.

REFERENCES

PART TWO — CHAPTER FIVE:
"The Foundations of Metabolic Therapy"

1. McKeown, Thomas, "What Determines a Society's Health?" *Journal of the Nutritional Academy,* Vol. I, No. I, Eugene, Oregon, 1970, p. 19.
2. Grossinger, Richard, *Planet Medicine,* Doubleday, N.Y., 1980, p. 116.
3. Grossinger, p. 76.
4. Grossinger, p. 77-90.
5. Grossinger, p. 63.
6. Lucas, Richard, *Nature's Medicine,* Parker Publishing Co., West Nyack, N.Y., 1966, p. 13.
7. Grossinger, p. 149.
8. Grossinger, p. 117.
9. Grossinger, p. 151.
10. Grossinger, p. 153.
11. Grossinger, p. 152.
12. Grossinger, p. 153-155.
13. Sobel, David, *Ways of Health,* Harcourt, Bruce, Jovanovich, N.Y., 1979, p. 33.
14. Grossinger, p. 225.
15. Chowka, Peter Barry, "The Drugging of America," *Journal of the Nutritional Academy,* Vol. II, No. I, 1978, Eugene, Oregon, p. 47.
16. Chowka, "The Drugging of America," p. 47.
17. Chowka, "The Drugging of America," p. 47.
18. Densmore, Emmet, M.D., *How Nature Cures,* Stillman and Co., N.Y., 1892, p. 15-45.
19. Chowka, Peter Barry, The Failure of Specialty Medicine," *Journal of the Nutritional Academy,* Vol. II, No. II, Eugene, Oregon, 1978, p. 64.
20. Mendelsohn, Peter, M.D., *Confessions for a Medical Heretic,* Warner Books, N.Y., 1979, p. 91-115.
21. Chowka, Peter Barry, "The Failure of Specialty Medicine," p. 64.
22. Ehrenreich, *The American Health Empire,* Random House, N.Y., 1971, p. 30.
23. Chowka, "The Drugging of America," p. 45.
24. Kotelchuck, David, *Prognosis Negative,* Random House, N.Y., 1976, p. 107.
25. Chowka, Peter Barry, "The Failure of Specialty Medicine," p. 45.
26. Morris, Nat, *The Cancer Blackout,* Regent House, Los Angeles, 1977, p. 27.
27. Morris, Nat, *The Cancer Blackout,* p. 33.
28. Morris, p. 43.
29. Morris, p. 47.

PART TWO — CHAPTER SIX:
"What Really Causes Cancer"

1. Ewan Cameron, Linus Pauling, *Cancer and Vitamin C,* Linus Pauling Institute of Science and Medicine, Menlo Park, CA, 1979, p. 4.
2. Israel, Lucien, M.D. *Conquering Cancer,* Random House, N.Y., 1979, p. 19, 20.
3. McKee, Dwight, M.D., "Dr. Livingston's Therapy," unpublished manuscript, 1981, p. 4.
4. Ibid., p. 4.
5. Agran, Larry, *The Cancer Connection,* Houghton Mifflin Co., Boston, 1977, p. 22-23.
6. Goodfield, June, *The Siege of Cancer,* Random House, N.Y., 1975, p. 99.
7. Pauling, *Cancer and Vitamin C,* p. 14.
8. Pauling, *Cancer and Vitamin C,* p. 10-12.
9. "Smoking and Health," a report of the U.S. Surgeon General, Washington, D.C., p. 2.
10. Germann, Donald R., M.D., *The Anti-Cancer Diet,* Wyden Books, N.Y., 1977, p. 46.
11. Germann, Donald R., M.D., The Anti-Cancer Diet, p. 46-47.
12. Whelan, Elizabeth, Ph.D., *Preventing Cancer,* W. W. Norton and Co., Inc., N.Y., 1970, p. 152-173.
13. "Cancer Rates and Risks," U.S. Department of Health, Education and Welfare, Washington, D.C., 1980, p. 5.
14. Hearings Before the Subcommittee on Nutrition, of the Committee on Agriculture, Nutrition and Forestry, United States Senate, June 12 and 13, 1978, U.S. Government Printing Office, Washington, D.C., 1978.
15. "Smoking and Health," a report of the U.S. Surgeon General.
16. "Cancer Rates and Risks," H.E.W., p. 5.
17. McGee, Charles, M.D., *How to Survive Modern Technology,* Ecology Press, Alamo, CA, 1979, p. 120.
18. Agran, Larry, *The Cancer Connection,* p. 174-177.
19. McGee, Charles, M.D., *How to Survive Modern Technology,* p. 122.
20. Agran, *The Cancer Connection,* p. 93.
21. McGee, *How to Survive Modern Technology,* p. 125.
22. Moss, Ralph, *The Cancer Syndrome,* Grove Press and Random House, N.Y., 1980, p. 187.
23. Fahey, John, M.D., "Cancer and Immune Response," *Journal of the Nutritional Academy,* Eugene, OR, 1979, p. 38.
24. Goodfield, *The Siege of Cancer,* p. 117.
25. Moss, Ralph, *The Cancer Syndrome,* p. 187.
26. Goodfield, June, *The Siege of Cancer,* p. 118.
27. Fahey, John, M.D., "Cancer and the Immune Response," p. 84.
28. Glassner, Ronald, M.D., *The Body Is Hero,* Random House, N.Y., 1976, p. 210.
29. Glassner, Ronald, M.D., *The Body Is Hero,* p. 210.
30. Hearings before the Subcommittee on Nutrition, p. 42.

31. Null, Gary, *The New Vegetarian,* p. 173.
32. Davis, Adelle, *Let's Get Well* quoted in Berkley, *Cancer,* p. 138.
33. Mindell, Earl, *The Vitamin Bible,* Rawson-Wade Publishers Inc., N.Y., 1979, p. 53.
34. Berkley, George, Ph.D., *Cancer,* p. 160.
35. Stauth, Cameron, "Caution: Poison," *Journal of the Nutritional Academy,* Eugene, OR, Fall, 1978, p. 25.
36. Stauth, Cameron, "Caution: Poison," *Journal of the Nutritional Academy,* p. 24.
37. Stauth, "Caution: Poison," p. 24.
38. Stauth, "Caution: Poison," p. 24.
39. Mae, Eydie, *How I Conquered Cancer Naturally,* with Chris Loeffler, Production House, San Diego, 1975, p. 110.

PART TWO — CHAPTER SEVEN:

"Cancer's 'Subtle Signals' That Can Save Your Life"

1. Moss, Ralph, *The Cancer Syndrome,* p. 28.
2. Berkley, George, Ph.D., *Cancer,* Prentice-Hall, Englewood Cliffs, NJ, 1978, p. 132.
3. Berkley, George, Ph.D., *Cancer,* p. 132.
4. Pauling, Linus and Cameron, Ewing, *Cancer and Vitamin C,* p. 6.
5. Brody, Jane E., *You Can Fight Cancer and Win,* McGraw-Hill, N.Y., 1978, p. 54.
6. R. Bangle, M. Berger, M. Levin, "Variations in the Morphogenesis of Squamous Carcinoma of the Cervix," *Cancer,* 1963, 1151-1159.
7. Cairns, John, *Cancer and Society,* W. H. Freeman and Co., San Francisco, 1978, p. 151.
8. Strax, Philip, M.D., *Early Detection,* Harper and Row, N.Y., 1974, p. 13.
9. Strax, Philip, M.D., *Early Detection,* p. 18.
10. Strax, Philip, M.D., *Early Detection,* p. 55.
11. Rosenbaum, Ruth, "Why America Is Losing the War on Cancer," *Journal of the Nutritional Academy,* April 1978, p. 14.
12. Rosenbaum, Ruth, "Why America Is Losing the War on Cancer," p. 14.
13. Rosenbaum, Ruth, "Why America Is Losing the War on Cancer," p. 14.
14. *Science,* July 13, 1979, quoted in Moss, *The Cancer Syndrome.*
15. *Rubin, Philip, Clinical Oncology for Medical Students and Physicians,* University of Rochester and American Cancer Society, N.Y., 1971, quoted in Moss, *The Cancer Syndrome,* p. 47.
16. Rubin, Philip, *Clinical Oncology for Medical Students and Physicians,* Moss, p. 40.
17. Berkley, George, Ph.D., *Cancer,* p. 131.
18. McKean, Kevin, "Chest X-Rays at Times Moot," *Portland Oregonian,* Nov. 20, 1980, p. A-12.
19. McKean, Kevin, "Chest X-Rays at Times Moot."
20. Brody, Jane, E., *You Can Fight Cancer and Win,* p. 74.
21. Pauling, Linus, *Cancer and Vitamin C,* p. 28.
22. Brody, Jane, *You Can Fight Cancer and Win,* p. 52.
23. McKean, Kevin, "Chest X-Rays at Times Moot," *Portland Oregonian.*
24. Moss, Ralph, *The Cancer Syndrome,* p. 27.
25. Whelan, Elizabeth, *Preventing Cancer,* p. 27.
26. Agran, Larry, *The Cancer Connection,* p. 25.
27. Agran, Larry, *The Cancer Connection,* p. 26.
28. *Freedom from Cancer,* Richardson, John, M.D., p. 183.

PART TWO — CHAPTER EIGHT:

"The Common Therapies: Positive and Negative Aspects"

1. Byrd, Benjamin, M.D., *American Legion,* quoted in Chowka, Peter Barry, "The Cancer Charity Ripoff," *East West Journal,* Boston, July 1978, p. 24.
2. *Encyclopedia Brittanica,* Fifteenth Edition, Volume 3, p. 766.
3. "Cancer Facts and Figures, 1980," American Cancer Society, N.Y., 1980, p. 7.
4. Epstein, Samuel, M.D., *The Politics of Cancer,* p. 328.
5. Epstein, Samuel, M.D., *The Politics of Cancer,* p. 329.
6. Chowka, Peter Barry, "The Cancer Charity Ripoff," p. 24.
7. Greenberg, Dan, "Cancer; Now the Bad News," *Washington Post,* January 19, 1975, quoted in Epstein, *The Politics of Cancer.*
8. *Textbook of Medical Surgical Nursing,* p. 873, also statement by Dr. Frank Rauscher of National Cancer Institute at White House Conference, May 5, 1972, and Dr. Charles Moertel of Mayo Clinic before National Cancer Institute, May 18, 1972.
9. Rosenbaum, Ruth, "Why America Is Losing the War on Cancer," *Journal of the Nutritional Academy,* p. 17.
10. Rosenbaum, Ruth, "Why America Is Losing the War on Cancer," p. 17.
11. Israel, Lucien, *Conquering Cancer,* p. 80.
12. Rosenbaum, Ruth, "Why America Is Losing the War on Cancer," p. 17.
13. Rosenbaum, Ruth, "Why America Is Losing the War on Cancer," p. 17.
14. Chowka, Peter Barry, "The Cancer Charity Ripoff," p. 24.
15. Chowka, Peter Barry, "The Cancer Charity Ripoff, p. 24.
16. Israel, Lucien, M.D., *Conquering Cancer,* p. 79.
17. Moss, Ralph, *The Cancer Syndrome,* p. 49.
18. Israel, Lucien, M.D., *Conquering Cancer,* p. 81.
19. Israel, Lucien, M.D., *Conquering Cancer,* p. 81.
20. Israel, Lucien, M.D., *Conquering Cancer,* p. 81.
21. Crile, George, M.D., *What Women Should Know about the Breast Cancer Controversy, Pocket Books, N.Y., 1974, p. 1-15.*
22. *Israel, Lucien, M.D., Conquering Cancer,* p. 93-94.
23. Bross, Irwin, D.J., Roswell Park Memorial Institute, in correspondence to Ralph Moss, quoted in *The Cancer Syndrome,* p. 52.
24. Moss, Ralph, *The Cancer Syndrome,* p. 53.
25. Israel, Lucien, M.D., *Conquering Cancer,* p. 95.
26. Moss, Ralph, *The Cancer Syndrome,* p. 65.
27. Richards, Victor, *Cancer, The Wayward Cell: Its Origins, Nature and Treatment,* U. of California Press, Berkeley, 1972, quoted in Moss, p. 69.
28. Richards, Victor, *Cancer, the Wayward Cell: Its Origins, Nature and Treatment,* quoted in Moss, p. 69.
29. Israel, Lucien, M.D., *Conquering Cancer,* p. 116.
30. Israel, Lucien, M.D., *Conquering Cancer,* p. 141.
31. Rosenbaum, Ruth, "Why America Is Losing the War on Cancer," p. 13.
32. Moss, Ralph, *The Cancer Syndrome,* p. 42.
33. Moss, Ralph, *The Cancer Syndrome,* p. 42.
34. Moss, Ralph, *The Cancer Syndrome,* p. 48.
35. Israel, Lucien, M.D., *Conquering Cancer,* p. 95.
36. Israel, Lucien, M.D., *Conquering Cancer,* p. 97.
37. Moss, Ralph, *The Cancer Syndrome,* p. 65.
38. Drummond, Hugh, M.D., "Pocketa Pocketa Machines," *Mother Jones,* January 1978, San Francisco.

39. Moss, Ralph, *The Cancer Syndrome,* p. 61.
40. *New York State Journal of Medicine,* March 1971, p. 554.
41. Moss, *The Cancer Syndrome,* p. 69.
42. Moss, *The Cancer Syndrome,* p. 66.
43. Crile, *What Women Should Know about the Breast Cancer Controversy,* Chapter 2.
44. *New York Times,* April 8, 1954, quoted in Moss, p. 58.

PART THREE — CHAPTER TEN:
"Individualizing the Anti-Cancer Program"

1. Williams, Roger, Ph.D., "Nutritional Individuality," *Journal of the Nutritional Academy,* Vol. II, No. II, Eugene, Oregon, 1978, p. 9.
2. Stauth, Cameron, "Applying Nutritional Individuality," *Journal of the Nutritional Academy,* Vol. II, No. II, Eugene, Oregon, 1978, p. 17.
3. Williams, Roger, Ph.D., "Nutritional Individuality," p. 10.

PART THREE — CHAPTER ELEVEN:
"The Anti-Cancer Diet"

1. Fry, Peggy, Ph.D., University of Texas Health Sciences Center, in statement to Hearings Before the Subcommittee on Nutrition, of the Committee on Agriculture, Nutrition and Forestry, United States Senate, June 12 and 13, 1978, U.S. Government Printing Office, Washington, D.C. p. 94.
2. Fry, Peggy, Ph.D., Hearings before Senate Subcommittee, p. 95.
3. Chowka, Peter Barry, "Lifting the Lid off a Fifty Year Coverup," *Journal of the Nutritional Academy,* Eugene, OR, 1978, p. 27.
4. Bayh, Marvella, Hearings before Senate Subcommittee, p. 97.
5. Cheraskin, E., M.D., D.M.D., Ringsdorf, W.M., D.M.D., Clark, J.W., D.D.S., *Diet and Disease,* Rodale Press, Emmaus, PA, 1968, p. 220.
6. Cheraskin, Ringsdorf, Clark, *Diet and Disease,* p. 221.
7. Pauling, Linus, Ph.D., and Cameron, Ewan, M.B., Ch. B., *Cancer and Vitamin C,* The Linus Pauling Institute of Science and Medicine, Menlo Park, CA, p. 111.
8. Cheraskin, Ringsdorf, Clark, *Diet and Disease,* p. 226.
9. Fry, Peggy, Ph.D., Hearings before Senate Subcommittee, p. 95.
10. Fry, Peggy, Ph.D., Hearings before Senate Subcommittee, p. 95.
11. Cheraskin, Ringsdorf, Clark, *Diet and Disease,* p. 227.
12. Cheraskin, Ringsdorf, Clark, *Diet and Disease,* p. 227.
13. McGee, Charles, M.D., *How to Survive Modern Technology,* Ecology Press, 1979, p. 49.
14. McGee, Charles, M.D., *How to Survive Modern Technology,* p. 49.
15. Germann, Donald, M.D., *The Anti-Cancer Diet,* Wyden Books, N.Y., 1977, p. 30.
16. Germann, Donald, M.D., *The Anti-Cancer Diet,* p. 82, 83.
17. Germann, Donald, M.D., *The Anti-Cancer Diet,* p. 30.
18. Kaslow, Arthur, M.D., and Miles, Richard, B., *Freedom From Chronic Disease,* J. P. Tarcher, L.A., 1979, p. 105.
19. Null, Gary, *The New Vegetarian,* William Morrow and Co., N.Y., 1978, p. 151-153.
20. Null, Gary, *The New Vegetarian,* p. 155.
21. Kloss, Jethro, *Back to Eden,* Woodbridge Press Publishing Co., Santa Barbara, CA, 1972, from the original edition of 1939, p. 68.

22. Kloss, Jethro, *Back to Eden,* p. 68.
23. Kloss, Jethro, *Back to Eden,* p. 69.
24. Null, Gary, *The New Vegetarian,* p. 161.
25. Livingston, Virginia, M.D. and Wheeler, Owen, M.D., *Food Alive,* the Livingston Wheeler Medical Clinic, San Diego, 1977, p. 67.
26. Livingston, Virginia, M.D., and Wheeler, Owen, M.D., *Food Alive,* p. 68.
27. Gerson, Max, M.D., *A Cancer Therapy,* p. 143.
28. Null, Gary, *The New Vegetarian,* p. 169.
29. Null, Gary, *The New Vegetarian,* p. 169.
30. Null, Gary, *The New Vegetarian,* p. 179.

PART THREE — CHAPTER TWELVE:
"The Power of Food Supplements"

1. Hueper, W. C., "Environmental Carcinogenesis in Man and Animals," *Annals of the New York Academy of Science,* New York, 108, Article 3, November 4, 1963.
2. McGee, Charles, M.D., *How to Survive Modern Technology,* Ecology Press, Alamo, CA, 1979, p. 45.
3. Turner, James, *The Chemical Feast,* Grossman Publishers, N.Y., 1970. p. 59.
4. McGee, p. 49.
5. Vallance, S., "Relationships Between Ascorbic Acid and Serum Proteins of the Immune System," *British Medical Journal,* London, Vol. 2, 1977, p. 437-438.
6. Passwater, Richard A., Ph.D., *Cancer and Its Nutritional Therapies,* Keats Publishing, New Canaan, CT, 1978, p. 120.
7. Pauling, Linus, Ph.D., and Cameron, Ewan, M. B., *Cancer and Vitamin C,* The Linus Pauling Institute of Science and Medicine, Menlo Park, CA, 1979, p. 109.
8. Passwater, p. 120.
9. Pauling, p. 110.
10. Pauling, p. 111.
11. Pauling, p. 115.
12. Berkley, George, Ph.D., *Cancer,* Prentice-Hall, Englewood Cliffs, NJ, 1978, p. 55.
13. Berkley, p. 55.
14. Passwater, p. 108.
15. Passwater, p. 123.
16. Warren, F. L., *Biochemistry Journal,* No. 37, 1943, p. 338-341.
17. Passwater, p. 123.
18. Passwater, p. 123.
19. Passwater, p. 124.
20. Pauling, p. 117.
21. Upton, Arthur, M.D., statement to "Hearings before Subcommittee on Agriculture, Nutrition and Forestry, U.S. Senate, June 12, 13, 1978, U.S. Government Printing Office, p. 42.
22. Upton, p. 43.
23. "Diet, Nutrition and Cancer Programs," National Cancer Institute, Washington, D.C., September 1977, p. 24.
24. Passwater, p. 104.
25. Passwater, p. 104.
26. Passwater, p. 105.

27. Berkley, p. 59.
28. Berkley, p. 59.
29. Germann, p. 87.
30. Passwater, p. 118.
31. Pauling, p. 114.
32. Passwater, p. 118
33. Passwater, p. 96.
34. Passwater, p. 97.
35. Passwater, p. 98.
36. Passwater, p. 98.
37. Passwater, p. 99, 103.
38. Wolf, Max, M.D., and Ransberger, Karl, Ph.D., *Enzyme Therapy,* Regent House, Los Angeles, 1972, p. 135.
39. Wolf and Ransberger, p. 141-142.
40. Wolf and Ransberger, p. 172.
41. Rolf and Ransberger, p. 171.
42. Manner, Harold, Ph.D., *The Death of Cancer,* Advanced Century Publishing Co, Chicago, 1978, p. 90.
43. Manner, p. 21.
44. Manner, p. 93.
45. Manner, p. 92-94.
46. Stauth, Cameron, "Alternative Cancer Therapies," *New Age,* July 1978, Brookline Village, MA, p. 35.
47. Passwater, p. 108-115.
48. Passwater, p. 110.
49. Passwater, p. 111-115.
50. Passwater, p. 117.
51. Passwater, p. 118.
52. Passwater, p. 106.
53. Passwater, p. 106.
54. Passwater, p. 106.
55. Cheraskin, E., M.D.; Ringsdorf, W. M., D.M.D.; Clark, J. W., D.D.S., *Diet and Disease,* Keats Publishing Inc., New Canaan, CT, 1968, p. 225.
56. Ibid, p. 225.
57. Berkley, p. 52.
58. Berkley, p. 53.
59. Berkley, p. 53.
60. Berkley, p. 72.
61. Holub, William, Ph.D., "Holism in Nutrition," *Journal of the Nutritional Academy,* Eugene, OR, Vol. II, No. III, p. 41-43.
62. Turner, p. 41.
63. Barnett, Stephen, M.D., and Gilda Knight, *The Health Robbers,* George F. Stickley, Co., Philadelphia, p. 23.

PART THREE — CHAPTER THIRTEEN:
"The Importance of Detoxification"

1. Bradford, Robert, *Now That You Have Cancer,* Choice Publications, Inc., Los Altos, CA, 1977, p. 61.
2. McGee, Charles, M.D., *How to Survive Modern Technology,* Ecology Press, Alama, CA, 1979, p. 50.
3. Ibid., p. 127-128.

4. Rona, Luanne, M.D., *Total Glow*. Enterprise Publishing, 1979, p. 125-126.
5. Agran, Larry, *The Cancer Connection,* Houghton Miflin Co., Boston, 1977, p. 93.
6. Ibid., p. 97.
7. Ibid., p. 96.
8. "Job Sites Unsafe," *Portland Oregonian,* October 20, 1980, p. A15.
9. McGee, p. 122.
10. Greenstein, Jesse, *Biochemistry of Cancer,* 1954, p. 509, quoted in Gerson, Max, M.D., *A Cancer Therapy,* Totality Books, Del Mar, CA, 1958, p. 72.
11. Gerson, Max, M.D., *A Cancer Therapy*. Totality Books, Del Mar, CA, 1958, p. 72.
12. Ibid., p. 72.
13. Greenstein, p. 513, in Gerson, p. 73.
14. Gerson, p. 137.
15. Ibid., p. 82.
16. Ibid., p. 190-191.
17. Passwater, Richard, Ph.D., *Cancer and Its Nutritional Therapies,* Keats, Publishing, Inc., New Canaan, CT, 1978, p. 154.
18. Rona, Luanne, M.D., *Total Glow,* p. 134.
19. Bricklin, Mark, *Natural Healing,* Rodale Press, Emmaus, PA, 1976, p. 305.
20. Buchman, Dia, *Water Therapy,* E. P. Dutton, New York, 1979, p. 4.
21. Buchman, p. 13.
22. Rona, Luanne, M.D., p. 132-133.
23. Ehret, Arnold, Prof., *The Mucusless Diet Healing System,* Ehret Literature Publishing Co., Beaumont, CA, 1977, p. 35.
24. Ehret, p. 35.
25. Interview, Barbara Poe, R.N., Eugene, Oregon, Feb. 5, 1981.
26. Mae, Eydie, *How I Conquered Cancer Naturally,* Production House, San Diego, 1975, p. 66.
27. Jensen, Bernard, D.C., N.D., *Nature Has a Remedy,* Escondido, CA, 1978, p. 74.
28. Goldstein, Jack, D.P.M., *Triumph Over Disease by Fasting,* Arco Publishing Co., New York, 1978, p. 200.
29. Goldstein, p. 200.
30. Jensen, p. 67.
31. Kaslow, Arthur, M.D., *Freedom from Chronic Disease,* J. P. Tarcher, Los Angeles, 1979, p. 96.

PART THREE — CHAPTER FOURTEEN:
"Structural Therapy and Cancer"

1. Koren, Tedd, Jr., "Cancer and Chiropractic," *The American Chiropractor,* Erie, PA, Vol. I, No. I., 1978, p. 18.
2. Ibid., p. 18.
3. Dintenfass, Julius, D.C., "The Clinical Significance of Chiropractic," *Journal of Energy Medicine,* North Miami, FL, Vol. I, No. I., p. 21.
4. Mason, John, Jr., "Perspectives in Biology and Medicine," Vol. 17, #3, 1974, quoted in Dintenfass, p. 21.
5. Dintenfass, p. 21.

6. Adams, Nevil, "Structural Integrity is a Health Necessity," *Journal of the Nutritional Academy,* Vol. II, No. III, Eugene, OR, p. 72.
7. Whigman, Jerry, D.C., "A Plausible Etiology for the High Incidence of Uterine Carcinoma in the Black Female," *Digest of Chiropractic Economics,* Vol. 22, No. 3, Farmington Hills, MI, p. 68.
8. Stauth, Cameron, "Spinal Stress," *Journal of the Nutritional Academy,* Eugene, OR, Vol. II, No. I, p. 17.
9. Ibid., p. 17.
10. Ibid., p. 17.
11. Ibid., p. 17.
12. Ibid., p. 19.
13. Ibid., p. 20.
14. Dintenfass, p. 23.
15. Gallo, Nick, "The New Age of Structural Therapy," *Journal of the Nutritional Academy,* Eugene, OR, Vol. II, No. I, p. 25.
16. Adams, p. 78.
17. Gallo, p. 27.
18. Koren, p. 19.
19. Simons, Victoria, D.C., "Chiropractic," *Health for the Whole Person,* Westview Press, Boulder, CO, 1980, p. 227.
20. Ibid., p. 228.
21. Frager, Robert, Ph.D., "Touch, Working with the Body," *Health for the Whole Person,* Westview Press, Boulder, CO, 1980, p. 227.
22. Ibid., p. 229.
23. Ibid., p. 212.
24. Ibid., p. 213.
25. Ibid., p. 214.
26. Stauth, Cameron, "M.E.A.," *Journal of the Nutritional Academy,* Vol. II, No. I, p. 11.
27. Ibid., p. 12.
28. Ibid., p. 12.

PART THREE — CHAPTER FIFTEEN:

"The Emotional and Spiritual Aspects of Cancer"

1. LeShan, Lawrence, Ph.D., *You Can Fight for Your Life,* M. Evans and Co., N.Y., 1977, p. 91.
2. Paget, Sir James, *Surgical Pathology,* Longman's Green, London, 1970, quoted in LeShan, p. 92.
3. Walshe, W. A., *The Nature and Treatment of Cancer,* Taylor and Walton, London, 1846.
4. Snow, H., *Clinical Notes on Cancer,* J. and A. Churchill, London, 1883.
5. Stauth, Cameron, "The Mind and Malignancy," *Journal of the Nutritional Academy,* Eugene, OR, Vol. I, No. I, 1970, p. 8.
6. Simonton, O. Carl, M.D.; Stephanie Matthews-Simonton; James Creighton, *Getting Well Again,* J. P. Tarcher, Inc., Los Angeles, 1978, p. 34.
7. Simonton and others, *Getting Well Again,* p. 50.
8. LaBarba, R. C., "Experimental and Environmental Factors in Cancer," *Psychosomatic Medicine,* 1970, p. 259.
9. Simonton and others, *Getting Well Again,* p. 44-46.
10. "Cancer and Worry Linked," *Portland Oregonian,* January 1978, p. A-22.
11. LeShan, Lawrence, *You Can Fight for Your Life,* p. 18-27.

12. Simonton and others, *Getting Well Again,* p. 60.
13. Ibid., p. 61.
14. Ibid., p. 62.
15. Ibid., p. 61.
16. Wheeler, J. I., and Caldwell, B.M., "Psychological Evaluation of Women with Cancer of the Breast and Cervix," *Psychosomatic Medicine,* 1955, p. 256-68.
17. LeShan, *You Can Fight for Your Life,* p. 12.
18. Simonton and others, *Getting Well Again,* p. 27-29.
19. Ibid., p. 6-8.
20. Ibid., p. 121-124.
21. Ibid., p. 86.
22. Ibid., p. 229.
23. Ibid., p. 114-116.
24. Ibid., p. 114-116.
25. Ibid., p. 114-116.
26. Ibid., p. 11.
27. Ibid., p. 10.
28. Morton, Bill, interview, Ft. Worth, Texas, December 1977.
29. Holzer, Hans, *Beyond Medicine,* Ballantine Books, N.Y., 1973, p. 85.
30. Ibid, p. 85.
31. Ibid., p. 85.
32. Ibid, p. 100.
33. Jaffe, Dennis, Ph.D., *Healing from Within,* Alfred A. Knopf, N.Y., 1980, p. 27.
34. McKechnie, Robert, M.D., *Strong Medicine,* J. J. Douglas, Ltd., Vancouver, B.C., 1972, p. 4.
35. Ibid., p. 4.
36. Mae, Eydie, *How I Conquered Cancer Naturally,* with Chris Loefler, Production House, San Diego, 1975, p. 196.
37. Ibid., p. 197.
38. Deverell, Dore, *How I Healed My Cancer Holistically,* published by Dore Deverell, 1978, p. 162.
39. Bloomfield, Harold, M.D., *The Holistic Way to Health and Happiness,* Simon and Schuster, N.Y., 1978, p. 257-259.

PART THREE — CHAPTER SIXTEEN:
"The Anti-Cancer Lifestyle"

1. Whelan, Elizabeth, *Preventing Cancer,* W. W. Norton and Co., N.Y., 1977, p. 27.
2. Ibid., p. 9.
3. Pearce, Joseph C., *Exploring the Crack in the Cosmic Egg,* quoted in Kaslow, *Freedom from Chronic Disease,* J. P. Tarcher, Los Angeles, 1980, p. 37.
4. Keleman, Stanley, D.C., *Somatic Reality,* Center Press, Berkeley, CA, 1979, p. 117.
5. Simonton, O. Carl, M.D., *Getting Well Again,* J. P. Tarcher, Los Angeles, 1978, p. 208.
6. Ibid., p. 209.
7. Ibid., p. 209.
8. Ibid., p. 209.
9. Ibid., p. 210.

10. Ardell, Donald B., "The Physical Disciplines and Health," *Health and the Whole Person,* Westview Press, Boulder, CO, 1980, p. 199.
11. Ibid., p. 199.
12. Ibid., p. 199.
13. Ibid., p. 198.
14. Ibid., p. 197.
15. Kaslow, Arthur, M.D., *Freedom from Chronic Disease,* J. P. Tarcher, Los Angeles, 1979, p. 96.
16. Ibid., p. 97.
17. Berkley, George, Ph.D., *Cancer,* Prentice Hall, Englewood Cliffs, NJ, 1978, p. 124.
18. Simonton, p. 214.
19. Goldstein, Jack, D.C., *Triumph Over Disease by Fasting,* Arco Publishing Co., N.Y., 1978, p. 206.
20. Simonton, p. 213.
21. Berkley, p. 124.
22. Rona, Luanne, M.D., *Total Glow,* Enterprise Publishing Co., Wilmington, DE, 1978, p. 18.
23. Berkley, p. 122.
24. Bloomfield, Harold, M.D., and Kory, Robert, *Health and Happiness,* Simon and Schuster, N.Y., 1978, p. 276.
25. Ibid., p. 276.
26. *The Smoking Digest*, U.S. Dept. H.E.W., National Institutes of Health, Bethesda, Maryland, p. 57-59.
27. Ibid., p. 6.
28. Ibid., p. 6.
29. Ibid., p. 17.
30. Ibid., p. 17.
31. Ibid., p. 17.
32. Ibid., p. 18.
33. *Cancer Facts and Figures,* American Cancer Society, N.Y., 1980, p. 8-15.
34. Whelan, Elizabeth, Ph.D., *Preventing Cancer,* W. W. Norton and Co., N.Y., 1977, p. 51-70.
35. Ibid., p. 51-70.
36. Ibid., p. 51-70.
37. Ibid., p. 51-70.
38. *Smoking and Health,* a report of the Surgeon General, U.S. Dept. of H.E.W., Office on Smoking and Health, U.S. Govt. Printing Office, Washington, D.C., p. 16-5 to 16-4.
39. Ibid., p. 16-7 to 16-13.
40. Ibid., p. 16-19 to 16-16.
41. Ibid., p. 16-16 to 16-18.
42. Ibid., p. 16-18 to 18-19.
43. Ibid, p. 16-19.
44. Mae, Eydie, *How I Conquered Cancer Naturally,* Production House, San Diego, p. 56-73.
45. Deverell, Dore, *How I Healed My Cancer Holistically,* published by Dore Deverell, p. 112-132.

PART FOUR — CHAPTER SEVENTEEN:
"A Lifetime Change"

1. Israel, Lucien, M.D., *Conquering Cancer,* Random House, N.Y., 1978, p. 6.
2. Ibid., p. 7.
3. Ibid., p. 7.
4. Ibid., p. 7.
5. Ibid., p. 80.
6. Maugh, Thomas, and Marx, Jean, "Seeds of Destruction: The 'Science' Report on Cancer Research, Plenum Publishing Co., N.Y., 1975, reported in Moss, *The Cancer Syndrome.*
7. Moss, Ralph W., *The Cancer Syndrome,* Grove Press, N.Y., 1980, p. 65.
8. Ibid., p. 54.
9. Ibid., p. 54.
10. Ibid., p. 54.
11. Israel, p. 95.
12. Ibid., p. 95.
13. Ibid., p. 96.
14. Ibid., p. 96.
15. Moss, p. 61.
16. Griffin, G. Edward, *World Without Cancer,* American Media, Thousand Oaks, CA, 1974, p. 200.
17. Israel, p. 97.
18. Ibid., p. 96-97.
19. Ibid., p. 125.
20. Moss, p. 61.

PART FOUR — CHAPTER EIGHTEEN:
"Combining a Metabolic Program with the More Common Therapies"

1. Rhoads, Jonathan E., statement to "Hearings Before the Subcommittee on Health and Scientific Research," of the Committee on Labor and Human Resources, U.S. Senate, March 5 and 7, 1979, Washington, D.C., p. 189.
2. Berkley, George, Ph.D., *Cancer,* Prentice-Hall, Englewood Cliffs, NJ, 1978, p. 45
3. Ibid., p. 45.
4. Ibid., p. 46.
5. Prasad, Ananda, *Trace Elements in Human Health and Disease,* quoted in Adams, Ruth and Murray, Frank, *Zinc,* Larchmont Books, N.Y., 1978, p. 55.
6. Pauling, Linus, Ph.D., *Cancer and Vitamin C,* The Linus Pauling Institute of Science and Medicine, Menlo Park, CA, 1979, p. 190.
7. Ibid., p. 191.
8. Ibid., p. 191.
9. Ibid., p. 191.
10. Adams, Ruth and Murray, Frank, *Vitamin E,* Larchmont Books, N.Y., 1978, p. 29.
11. Pauling, p. 191.
12. Ibid., p. 192.

13. Berkley, p. 47.
14. Pauling, p. 193.
15. Pauling, p. 193.
16. Adams, Ruth and Murray, Frank, *Vitamin C,* Larchmont Books, N.Y., 1978, p. 107.
17. Adams, Ruth and Murray, Frank, *Vitamin E,* p. 23.
18. Ibid., p. 23.
19. Shute, Wilfrid, M.D., *Your Child and Vitamin E,* Keats Publishing Co., New Canaan, CT, 1979, p. 27.
20. Israel, Lucien, M.D., *Conquering Cancer,* Random House, N.Y., 1979, p. 140.
21. Ibid., 77-92.
22. Rhoads, Jonathan, M.D., "Hearings," p. 189.
23. "Food Stronger than Medicine?", *Journal of the Nutritional Academy,* Eugene, OR, Fall, 1978, p. 40.
24. Cheraskin, E., M.D.; Ringsdorf, W. M., D.M.D.; Clark, J. W., D.D.S., *Diet and Disease,* Keats Publishing Co., New Canaan, CT, 1968, p. 227.
25. Adams and Murray, *Vitamin E,* p. 27.

PART FOUR — CHAPTER NINETEEN:
"A Program for Other Diseases"

1. Grossinger, Richard, *Planet Medicine,* Anchor Press/Doubleday, N.Y., 1980, p. 116.
2. Dubos, Rene, *Ways of Health,* edited by David Sobel, Harcourt, Brace, Jovanovich, N.Y., 1979, p. 27, 28, 29, 31, 32.
3. Cheraskin, E., M.D.,; Ringsdorf, W. M., D.M.D.; Clark, J. W., D.D.S., *Diet and Disease,* Keats Publishing, Inc., New Canaan, CT, 1968, p. 88-292.
4. Ibid., p. 5, 6.
5. Williams, Roger, Ph.D., *Nutrition Against Disease,* Pitman Publishing Corp., N.Y., 1971, p. 1.
6. Rona, Luanne, M.D., *Total Glow,* Enterprise Publishing Co., Wilmington, DE, 1979, p. xvi.
7. Ibid., p. 3.
8. Gerson, Max, M.D., *A Cancer Therapy,* Totality Books, Del Mar, CA, 1958, p. 19.
9. Ibid., p. 20.
10. Chowka, Peter Barry, "The Failure of Specialty Medicine," *Journal of the Nutritional Academy,* Vol. II, No. II, p. 64.
11. Duenwald, Mary, "I Know How You Feel," *Journal of the Nutritional Academy,* Vol. II, No. III, p. 62.
12. Stauth, Cameron, "Applying Nutritional Individuality," *Journal of the Nutritional Academy,* Vol. II, No. II, p. 22.
13. Ibid., p. 22-23.
14. Ibid., p. 23.
15. Ibid., p. 24.
16. Stauth, Cameron, "Non-Specific Therapy," *Journal of the Nutritional Academy,* Eugene, OR, Vol. II, No. III, p. 25.
17. Ibid., p. 26.
18. Ibid., p. 26.

BIBLIOGRAPHY

Adams, Nevil, "Structural Therapy Is a Health Necessity," *Journal of the Nutritional Academy,* Vol. II, No. II, Eugene, OR, p. 72.

Adams, Ruth and Murray, Frank, *Improving Your Health With Zinc,* Larchmont Books, N.Y., 1978.

Adams, Ruth and Murray, Frank, *Improving Your Health With Vitamin C,* Larchmont Books, N.Y., 1978.

Adams, Ruth and Murray, Frank, *Improving Your Health With Vitamin E,* Larchmont Books, N.Y., 1978.

Agran, Larry, *The Cancer Connection,* Houghton Mifflin Co., Boston, 1977.

Agriculture, Nutrition and Forestry, Committee on, U.S. Senate, *Subcommittee on Nutrition, Hearings,* U.S. Govt. Printing Office, Washington, D.C., 1978.

American Cancer Society, *Cancer Facts and Figures,* 1980, N.Y., 1980. Also: 1976, 1977, 1978, 1979.

American Health Foundation, *Food and Nutrition Committee, Activities Report,* N.Y., 1978.

Ames, B. N., "Identifying Environmental Chemicals Causing Mutations and Cancer," *Science,* Washington, D.C., May 11, 1979, p. 587.

Barrett, Stephen, M.D., and Knight, Gilda, *The Health Robbers,* George F. Stickley Co., Philadelphia, 1976.

Barth, George F., *Nova Yoga,* New American Library, 1974.

Bauer, C. H., "Decrease of Human Serum Fucosyltransferase as an Indicator of Successful Tumor Therapy," *Science,* Washington, D.C., May 11, 1979, p. 647.

Benson, Herbert, M.D., *The Mind/Body Effect,* Simon and Schuster, N.Y., 1979.

Berkley, George E., *Cancer,* Prentice-Hall, Englewood Cliffs, NJ, 1978.

Bloomfield, Harold, M.D., and Kory, Robert, *Health and Happiness,* Simon and Schuster, N.Y., 1978.

Blot, William J., "Geography of Cancer," *Cancer News,* American Cancer Society, N.Y., Spring 1978, p. 18.

Boone, C. W., "Spontaneous Neoplastic Transformation in Vitro: A Form of Foreign Body Tumor Igenesis," *Science,* Washington, D.C., Ap. 13, 1979, p. 177.

Bosco, Dominick, "Nutrition Under the Knife," *Prevention,* Emmaus, PA, Jan. 1978, p. 83.

Boyle, Robert, *Malignant Neglect,* Alfred A. Knopf, N.Y., 1979.

Bradford, Robert W., with Culbert, Mike, *Now That You Have Cancer,* Choice Publications, Los Altos, CA, 1977.

Bricklin, Mark, *Natural Healing,* Rodale Press, Emmaus, PA, 1976.

Broad, W. J., "New Strength in the Diet-Disease Link?" *Science,* Washington, D.C., Nov. 9, 1979, p. 666.

Brody, Jane, with Holleb, Arthur, M.D., *You Can Fight Cancer and Win,* McGraw-Hill Book Co., N.Y., 1977.

Buchman, Dian Dincin, *Water Therapy,* E. P. Dutton, N.Y., 1979.

Burrows, N.E., "Cancer Safety Controversy," *New York Times Magazine,* N.Y., Mar. 25, 1979, p. 82.

Cairns, John, *Cancer, Science and Society,* W. H. Freeman and Co., San Francisco, 1978.

Cameron, Ewan and Pauling, Linus, *Cancer and Vitamin C,* The Linus Pauling Institute of Science and Medicine, Menlo Park, CA, 1979.

Cheraskin, E., M.D.; Ringsdorf, W. M., Jr., D.M.D.; and Clark, J. W., D.D.S., *Diet and Disease,* Keats Publishing Inc., New Canaan, CT, 1968.

Chowka, Peter Barry, "The Drugging of America," *Journal of the Nutritional Academy,* Vol. II, No. I, Eugene, OR, p. 44.

Chowka, Peter Barry, "Good News—We've Lost the War on Cancer," *Journal of the Nutritional Academy,* Vol. II, No. I, p. 66.

Chowka, Peter Barry, "The Failure of Specialty Medicine," *Journal of the Nutritional Academy,* Vol. II, No. III, Eugene, OR, p. 48.

Chowka, Peter Barry, "The New Food Consciousness," *New Age,* Brookline Village, MA, Dec., 1978, p. 30.

Chowka, Peter Barry, "Diet and Cancer," *Journal of the Nutritional Academy,* Vol. I, No. II, Eugene, OR, p. 29.

Chowka, Peter Barry, "The Cancer Charity Ripoff," *East West Journal,* Brookline, MA, July 1978, p. 22.

Chowka, Peter Barry, "Steve McQueen, Legacy of a Medical Outlaw," *New Age,* Jan. 1981, p. 28.

Clark, Randolph, M.D., Cumley, Russell, Ph.D., *The Year Book of Cancer 1970,* Year Book Medical Publishers, Chicago, 1970.

Cousins, Norman, "What I Learned from 3,000 Doctors," *Journal of the Nutritional Academy,* Vol. I, No. II, Eugene, OR, p. 11.

Council on Nutritional Research, *Nutritional Program,* Dallas, TX, Nov. 1966.

Culbert, Michael, *Freedom from Cancer,* Pocket Books, N.Y., 1976.

Crile, Georg, M.D., *What Women Should Know About the Breast Cancer Controversy,* Macmillan Publishing Co., N.Y., 1973.

Donahoe, P. K., "Mullerian Duct Regression in the Embryo Correlated with Cytoxic Activity Against Human Ovarian Cancer," *Science,* Washington, D.C., Aug. 31, 1979, p. 913.

Deverell, Dore, *How I Healed My Cancer Holistically,* 1978.

Dintenfass, Julius, D.C., "The Clinical Significance of Chiropractic," *Journal of Energy Medicine,* North Miami, FL, Vol. I, No. I, p. 20.

Drummond, Hugh, M.D., "Pocketa Pocketa Machines," *Mother Jones,* San Francisco, July 1978.

Dubos, Rene, Ph.D., "Bolstering the Body Against Disease," *Journal of the Nutritional Academy,* Vol. II, No. III, Eugene, OR, p. 54.

Duenwald, Mary, "Russell Bates Cares," *Journal of the Nutritional Academy,* Vol. II, No. III, Eugene, OR, p. 71.

Duenwald, Mary, "Research Doctors Blaze New Trails," *Journal of the Nutritional Academy,* Eugene, OR, Vol. II, No. III, p. 80.

Ehret, Arnold, *Mucusless Diet Healing System,* Erhet Literature Publishing Co., Beaumont, CA, 1922.

Eisenbud, M., "Environmental Causes of Cancer," *Environment,* Washington, D.C., Jan. 1979, p. 44.

Epstein, Samuel, M.D., *The Politics of Cancer,* Sierra Club Books, San Francisco, 1978.

Feltman, John, "Bran, Vitamin C and Cancer," *Prevention,* Emmaus, PA, Jan. 1978, p. 52.

Fearon, Douglas, M.D., Austen, Frank, M.D., "Current Concepts in Immunology," *New England Journal of Medicine,* Boston, MA, July 31, 1980, p. 259.

Fahey, John C., M.D., "Cancer and the Immune Response," *Journal of the Nutritional Academy,* Vol. II, No. III, Eugene, OR, p. 38.

Friedman, Meyer, M.D., and Rosenbaum, Ray, M.D., *Type A Behavior and Your Heart,* Fawcett Crest, N.Y., 1974.

Friedman, Milton, "Holistic Health, Is Washington Listening?", *Journal of the Nutritional Academy,* Vol. I, No. II, Eugene, OR, p. 41.

Gallo, Nick, "The New Age of Structrual Therapy," *Journal of the Nutritional Academy,* Vol. II, No. I, Eugene, OR, p. 24.

Germann, Donald, M.D., *The Anti-Cancer Diet,* Wyden Books, N.Y., 1977.

Gerson, Max, M.D., *A Cancer Therapy,* Totality Books, Del Mar, CA, 1958.

Glasser, Ronald, M.D., *The Greatest Battle,* Random House, N.Y., 1976.

Glasser, Ronald, M.D., *The Body Is Hero,* Random House, N.Y., 1976.

Goldstein, Jack, D.P.M., *Triumph Over Disease By Fasting,* Arco Publishing Co., N.Y., 1977.

Goodfield, June, *The Siege of Cancer,* Dell Publishing Co., N.Y., 1975.

Gori, Gio B., Ph.D., "Diet and Degenerative Disease," *Journal of the Nutritional Academy,* Vol. II, No. II, Eugene, OR, p. 50.

Griffin, G. Edward, *World Without Cancer,* American Media, Thousand Oaks, CA, 1974.

Grossinger, Richard, *Planet Medicine,* Anchor Books, Garden City, NY, 1980.

Haught, S. J., *Has Dr. Max Gerson A True Cancer Cure?,* London Press, North Hollywood, CA, 1962.

Henkoff, Ronald, "A Strange Sort of Therapy," *Newsweek,* Oct. 10, 1980, p. 65.

Health, Education and Welfare, U.S. Dept. of, *The Smoking Digest,* Public Health Service, Washington, D.C., 1977.

Health, Education and Welfare, U.S. Dept. of, *Cancer Rates and Risks,* Public Health Service, Washington, D.C., 1974.

Health, Education and Welfare, U.S. Dept. of, *Smoking and Health,* Public Health Service, 1979.

Health and Scientific Research, Subcommittee on, *Hearings,* Washington, D.C., March 5 and 7, 1979.

Health Policy Advisory Center, *The American Health Empire,* Random House, N.Y., 1971.

Hixson, Joseph, *Patchwork Mouse,* Anchor Press, N.Y., 1976.

Hoffer, Abram, Ph.D., and Walker, Morton, D.P.M., *Orthomolecular Nutrition,* Keats Publishing Co., New Canaan, CT, 1978.

Holzer, Hans, *Beyond Medicine,* Ballantine Books, N.Y., NY, 1973.

Holub, William R., Ph.D., "Holism in Nutritional Therapy," *Journal of the Nutritional Academy,* Eugene, OR, Vol. II, No. III, p. 41.

Israel, Lucien, M.D., *Conquering Cancer,* Random House, N.Y., 1978.

Jaffe, Dennis, Ph.D., *Healing From Within,* Alfred A. Knopf, N.Y., 1980.

Jensen, Bernard, D.C., *Nature Has a Remedy,* Escondido, CA, 1978.

Kaslow, Arthur, M.D., and Miles, Richard, *Freedom From Chronic Disease,* J. P. Tarcher, Los Angeles, 1979.

Keleman, Stanley, *Somatic Reality,* Center Press, Berkeley, CA, 1979.

Kloss, Jethro, *Back to Eden,* Woodbridge Press Publishing Co., Santa Barbara, CA, 1972.

Koren, Tedd, "Cancer and Chiropractic," *The American Chiropractor,* Erie, PA, Dec. 1978, p. 18.

Kulvinskas, Viktoras, M.S., *Survival Into the Twenty-First Century,* Omangod Press, Wethersfield, CT, 1975.

Komin, Richard, M.D., *Mega-Nutrition,* McGraw Hill, N.Y., 1980.

Kunz-Bircher, Ruth, *The Bircher-Benner Health Guide,* Woodbridge Press Publishing Co., Santa Barbara, CA, 1980.

LeShan, Lawrence, *You Can Fight For Your Life,* M. Evans and Co., N.Y., 1976.

Levitt, Paul M. and Guralnick, Elissa, *The Cancer Reference Book,* Paddington Press Ltd., N.Y., 1979.

Livingston, Virginia, M.D., *Cancer: A New Breakthrough,* Production House Publishers, San Diego, 1972.

Livingston, Virginia, M.D., and Wheeler, Owen, M.D., *Food Alive,* the Livingston-Wheeler Medical Clinic, San Diego, 1977.

Livingston, Virginia, M.D., and Wheeler, Owen, M.D., *Compendium,* The Livingston-Wheeler Medical Clinic, San Diego, 1977.

Lynch, Henry, *Cancer and You,* Charles C. Thomas, Publisher, Springfield, IL, 1971.

Mae, Eydie, *How I Conquered Cancer Naturally,* Production House, San Diego, 1975.

Maroon, Joseph, M.D., *What You Can Do About Cancer,* Doubleday and Co., N.Y., 1969.

McKechnie, Robert, M.D., *Strong Medicine,* J. J. Douglas Ltd., Vancouver, B.C., Canada, 1972.

McGee, Charles T., *How to Survive Modern Technology,* Ecology Press, Alamo, CA, 1979.

McGrady, Pat, *The Savage Cell,* Basic Books Inc., N.Y., 1964.

McKeown, Thomas, Ph.D., "What Determines a Society's Health?" *Journal of the Nutritional Academy,* Eugene, OR, Vol. I, No. II, p. 17.

Mendelsohn, Robert, M.D., *Confessions of a Medical Heretic,* Warner Books, N.Y., 1979.

Mindell, Earl, *Vitamin Bible,* Rawson-Wade Publishers, Inc., N.Y., 1979.

Montagna, Joseph, *People's Desk Reference,* Quest for Truth Publications, Inc., Lake Oswego, OR, 1979.

Morris, Nat, *The Cancer Blackout,* Regent House, Los Angeles, 1977.

Moss, Ralph, *The Cancer Syndrome,* Grove Press, N.Y., 1980.

National Cancer Institute, "Estimates of the Fraction of Cancer in the United States Related to Occupational Factors," Washington, D.C., 1978.

National Cancer Institute, "National Cancer Program," Washington, D.C., 1976.

National Cancer Institute, "Diet, Nutrition and Cancer Program," Washington, D.C., 1977.

Nicolson, G. L., "Cancer Metastasis," *Scientific American,* N.Y., March 1979, p. 66.

Nobile, Philip, *King Cancer,* Sheed and Ward, N.Y., 1975.

Null, Gary, *The New Vegetarian,* William Morrow and Co., N.Y., 1978.

Passwater, Richard, Ph.D., *Cancer and Its Nutritional Therapies,* Keats Publishing Inc., New Canaan, CT, 1978.

Popenoe, Cris, *Wellness,* Yes, Inc., Washington, D.C., 1977.

Rapaport, Stephen, *Strike Back at Cancer,* Prentice-Hall, Englewood Cliffs, NJ, 1978.

Richardson, John, M.D., *Laetrile Case Histories,* Bantam Books, N.Y., 1977.

Rona, Luanne, M.D., *Total Glow,* Enterprise Publishing Co., Wilmington, DE, 1979.

Rosenberg, Harold, *The Book of Vitamin Therapy,* Berkeley Publishing Corp., N.Y., 1974.

Scarf, Maggie, "Images that Heal," *Psychology Today,* N.Y., Sept. 1980, p. 32.

Rovera, G., "Induction of Differentiation in Human Promyelocytic Leukemia Cells by Tumor Promoters," *Science,* Washington, D.C., May 25, 1979, p. 868.

Shute, Wilfred, M.D., *Your Child and Vitamin E,* Keats Publishing Co., New Canaan, CT, 1979.

Simonton, O. Carl, M.D., and Matthews-Simonton, Stephanie and Creighton, James, *Getting Well Again,* J. P. Tarcher, Inc., Los Angeles, 1978.

Sobel, David, *Ways of Health,* Harcourt, Brace, Jovanouich, N.Y., 1979.

Stauth, Cameron, "Alternative Cancer Therapies," *New Age,* Brookline Village, MA, July 1978, p. 28.

Stauth, Cameron, "The Cancer Preventive Lifestyle," *New Age,* Brookline Village, MA, July 1978, p. 44.

Stauth, Cameron, "M.E.A." *Journal of the Nutritional Academy,* Eugene, OR, Vol. II, No. I, p. 8.

Stauth, Cameron, "Nutrition's Vital Role in Health," *Digest of Chiropractic Economics,* Vol. 21, No. 3, Farmington, Hills, MI, p. 76.

Stauth, Cameron, "Spinal Stress," *Journal of the Nutritional Academy,* Vol. II, No. I, Eugene, OR, p. 16.

Stauth, Cameron, "Applying Nutritional Individuality," *Journal of the Nutritional Academy,* Vol. II, No. II, Eugene, OR, p. 14.

Stauth, Cameron, "The Plowboy Interview," *Mother Earth News,* Issue No. 59, p. 17.

Stauth, Cameron, "Non-Specific Metabolic Therapy," *Journal of the Nutritional Academy,* Vol. II, No. III, p. 7.

Stauth, Cameron, "Steve McQueen, His Grim Battle," *People Magazine,* N.Y., Oct. 20, 1980, p. 50.

Stauth, Cameron, "Nutrition for Life," *New Age,* Brookline Village, MA, Dec. 1978, p. 46.

Stauth, Cameron, "The Biochemistry of Emotion," *Journal of Health Science,* Vol. I, No. I, Eugene, OR, p. 8.

Stauth, Cameron, "Dueling Porkers," *Saturday Evening Post,* Indianapolis, Feb. 1980.

Stauth, Lorraine, "Reversing the Irreversible, *Journal of the Nutritional Academy,* Vol. II, No. II, Eugene, OR, p. 60.

Stauth, Lorraine, "Recovering from Medical Maltreatment," *Journal of the Nutritional Academy,* Vol. II, No. II, p. 63.

Stone, Irwin, *The Healing Factor,* Grosset and Dunlap, N.Y., 1972.

Turner, James, *The Chemical Feast,* Grossman Publishers, N.Y., 1970.

Strax, Philip, M.D., *Early Detection,* Harper and Row, N.Y., 1974.

Wallin, Bernice, *I Beat Cancer,* Contemporary Books, Inc., Chicago, 1978.

Whelan, Elizabeth, Ph.D., *Preventing Cancer,* W. W. Norton and Co., N.Y., 1977.

Williams, Roger J., Ph.D., *Nutrition Against Disease,* Bantam Books, N.Y., 1971.

Williams, Roger J., Ph.D., *The Wonderful World Within You,* Bantam Books, N.Y., 1977.

Williams, Roger J., Ph.D., "Nutritional Individuality," *Journal of the Nutritional Academy,* Vol. II, No. II, Eugene, OR, p. 8.

Yatvin, M.B., "Hyperthermia and Local Anesthetics: Potentiation of Survival in Tumor-Bearing Mice," *Science,* Washington, D.C., July 13, 1979, p. 195.

Information on Doctors Using the Metabolic Approach to Cancer

The Cancer Education Association, an educational organization that dispenses information about cancer prevention and cancer therapy, will send you a fact sheet on doctors who apply non-toxic modalities in their work. The fact sheet will include names, addresses, telephone numbers, and a brief description of the approach of the doctors listed.

To receive this information, fill out the attached card and mail to: 1238 Hayes, Eugene, Oregon 97402.

☐ Please send me information about doctors who employ the metabolic approach to cancer.

____

(name) (phone)

____

(address)

____

(city, state, zip)